Julius Scott and the Importance of Being

Julius Scott and the Importance of Being

Elisha Renne

Maize Books

Published in the United States of America by
Michigan Publishing
Manufactured in the United States of America

DOI: http://doi.org/10.3998/mpub.14407025

ISBN 978-1-60785-871-3 (paper)
ISBN 978-1-60785-870-6 (open-access)

An imprint of Michigan Publishing, Maize Books serves the publishing needs of the University of Michigan community by making high-quality scholarship widely available in print and online. It represents a new model for authors seeking to share their work within and beyond the academy, offering streamlined selection, production, and distribution processes. Maize Books is intended as a complement to more formal modes of publication in a wide range of disciplinary areas.

http://www.maizebooks.org

Contents

Acknowledgments ~ vii

Chapter 1: Introduction ~ 1

Chapter 2: My Human, Julius ~ 13

Chapter 3: "Thank you, God, for My Own Bathroom": Elementary School Desegregation in Houston, Texas ~ 27

Chapter 4: Diabetes: The Dangerous Disease ~ 37

Chapter 5: *The Common Wind* ~ 59

Chapter 6: The Haitian Revolution and Isaac Sasportas's Jamaican Conspiracy ~ 77

Chapter 7: On Race ~ 97

Chapter 8: Memories and Memorials ~ 111

Bibliography ~ 127

Acknowledgments

The importance of documenting the life of Julius Scott was the impetus for writing this short biography, which reflects our meeting at the University of Michigan in 1999 and continued until his death in December 2021. I am grateful to his mother, Ann Scott, who explained aspects of his early childhood, his education, and his difficulties with type 1 diabetes. She also made corrections in the manuscript and provided many interesting photographs. I am grateful to others who read the manuscript draft, including Susan Bergh, Willard Brooks, Jim Chaffers, and Jim Leitzel. Thanks also to Kelly Askew who alerted me to Maize Books and to Ellen Bauerle, executive editor of the University of Michigan Press, who introduced me to the Maize Books Michigan Publishing Services Editorial Coordinator, Marisa Mercurio. Annie Carter, the Digital Publishing Coordinator for Maize Books at Michigan Publishing Services, has helpfully assisted me with digital work on the manuscript.

This volume focuses on Julius "Scotty" Scott and I've intentionally left myself out of its pages. Indeed, Julius is the main person who needs to be acknowledged and thanked, as bringing his interview remarks, his writing and teaching materials, photographs, and journal entries together has provided me with his presence, no matter how unfortunately ephemeral it has been.

Elisha Renne

Chapter 1
Introduction

"Just my luck," as Julius Scott put it when he was diagnosed with type 1 diabetes in 1973 at the beginning of his first year as an undergraduate at Brown University in Providence, Rhode Island. Yet, in 1977, he graduated *magna cum laude*, with honors in history, a reflection of his intellectual brilliance and the extensive support of his family, who valued education. Indeed, his grandfather, Julius S. Scott, Sr., was the ninth president of Wiley College in Marshall, Texas, from 1948 to 1958; his father, Julius S. Scott, Jr., was the fourteenth president, serving from 1996 to 1998; and his mother, Ianthia H. Scott (Ann) was a librarian who cherished books and instilled a love of reading in her son.

While Julius S. Scott III, or "Scotty" as his family knew him, did not serve as a college president, his significant scholarship was evidenced in his 1986 PhD dissertation, which was later published as *The Common Wind: Afro-American Currents in the Age of the Haitian Revolution* in 2018, widely regarded as a transformative contribution to Atlantic world history (Figure 1.1).

As was described in his *New York Times* obituary, Julius, through "his meticulous, imaginative and tenacious research, bolstered by his fluency in French and Spanish, revealed a previously undiscovered 18th-century intercontinental communication network" (Roberts 2021). Admiringly reviewed in many important journals, the book received several awards, which included the Museum of African American History Stone Book Award in 2019 and the Franz Fanon Book Award in 2020. These accolades came as a sort of compensation at the time of his worsening health, a consequence of diabetes. At the Zoom memorial, "Julius S. Scott: ¡Presente!," organized by his colleague and friend, Laurent Dubois, on December 13, 2021, people expressed their great

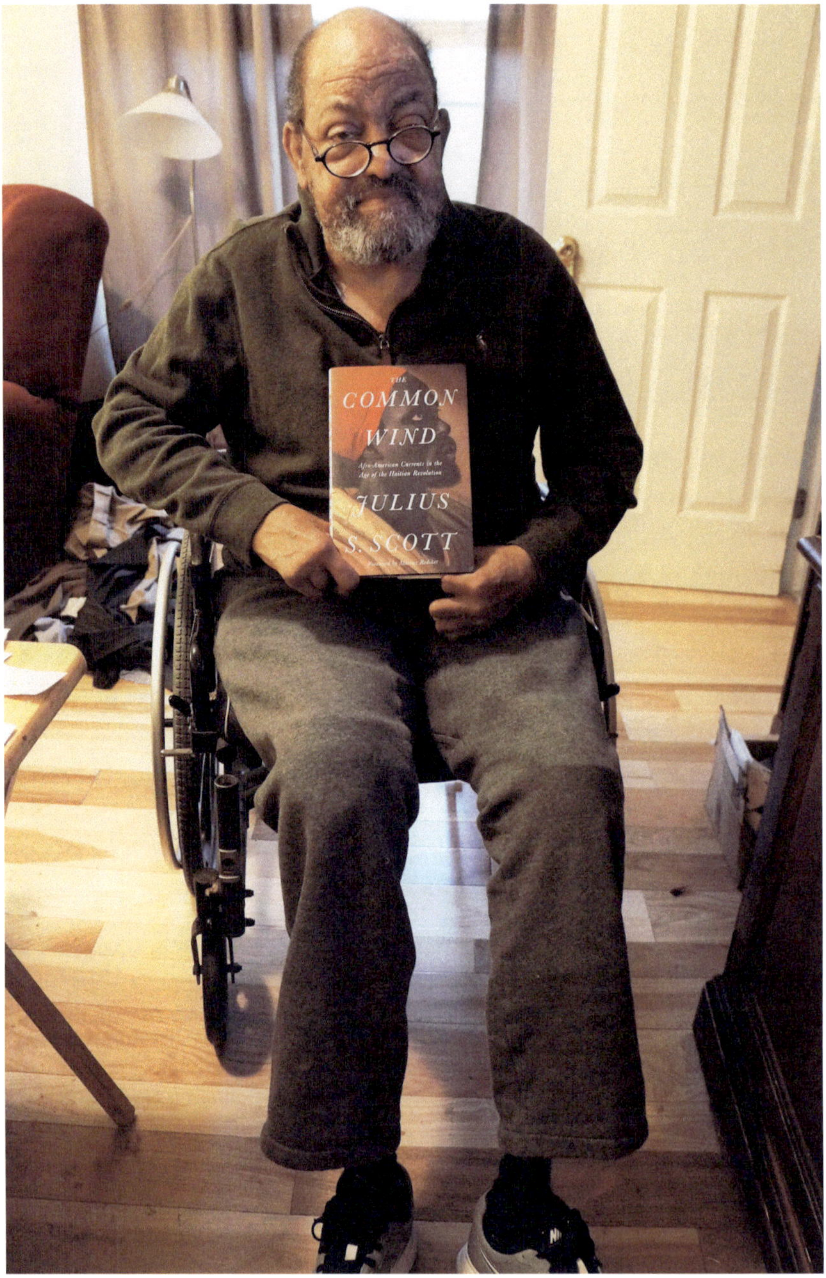

Figure 1.1. Julius Scott holding a copy of his book, *The Common Wind*, Ann Arbor, Michigan, November 9, 2018; photograph by E.P. Renne.

admiration for Julius's work, citing passages from *The Common Wind*, and conveyed their sadness that he had gone.[1]

This biographical endeavor is based on interviews with Julius and his family; his dissertation and book; his articles, book chapters, and syllabi; as well as my own journal entries on Julius's life, mainly from 1999 until his death on December 6, 2021. As is discussed in Chapter 3, when he was six years old, Julius was one of the first two Black children to integrate MacGregor Elementary School in Houston, Texas, in 1961 (Figure 1.2).

His parents expressed their support for his continuing at MacGregor by successfully pressuring the Houston school board to end the school's practice of segregated bathrooms. When the family later moved to Atlanta, they supported his attendance at the exclusive private school, Westminster, for his secondary school education. It was expensive, even with a financial assistance from the Methodist Church. So, when his father had news of the Stouffer Foundation that provided scholarships for African American students to attend segregated private schools, he encouraged Julius to apply. Julius passed the required Metropolitan Achievement Test, the standardized test used by the Stouffer Foundation, and was subsequently interviewed. He was then considered an appropriate recipient of a Stouffer Foundation scholarship.

On receiving this award, he and his father investigated the options available. The Indian Springs School, a private boarding school in Indian Springs Village, Shelby County, Alabama, seemed like a good fit for Julius. Since his father did not have time to take him to see other schools, plans were made for him to attend Indian Springs. Before classes began, however, he traveled to Duke University where he participated in the required ABC (A Better Chance) Program, which assisted students in transitioning from public (integrated) to private (all White) schools. Classes included several standard subjects such as English and math as well as study hall practices, watching movie classics, and sports (Purdy 2018: 126). In the fall, Julius began his classes at Indian Springs. He completed his education there in 1973.

Julius applied to several universities for his undergraduate study, including Brown and Harvard, and was accepted by all due to his good record at Indian

[1] This Zoom memorial program was co-sponsored by Conversations in Caribbean Studies, the Democracy Initiative and the Woodson Institute at the University of Virginia, and the #Slaveryarchive Book Club.

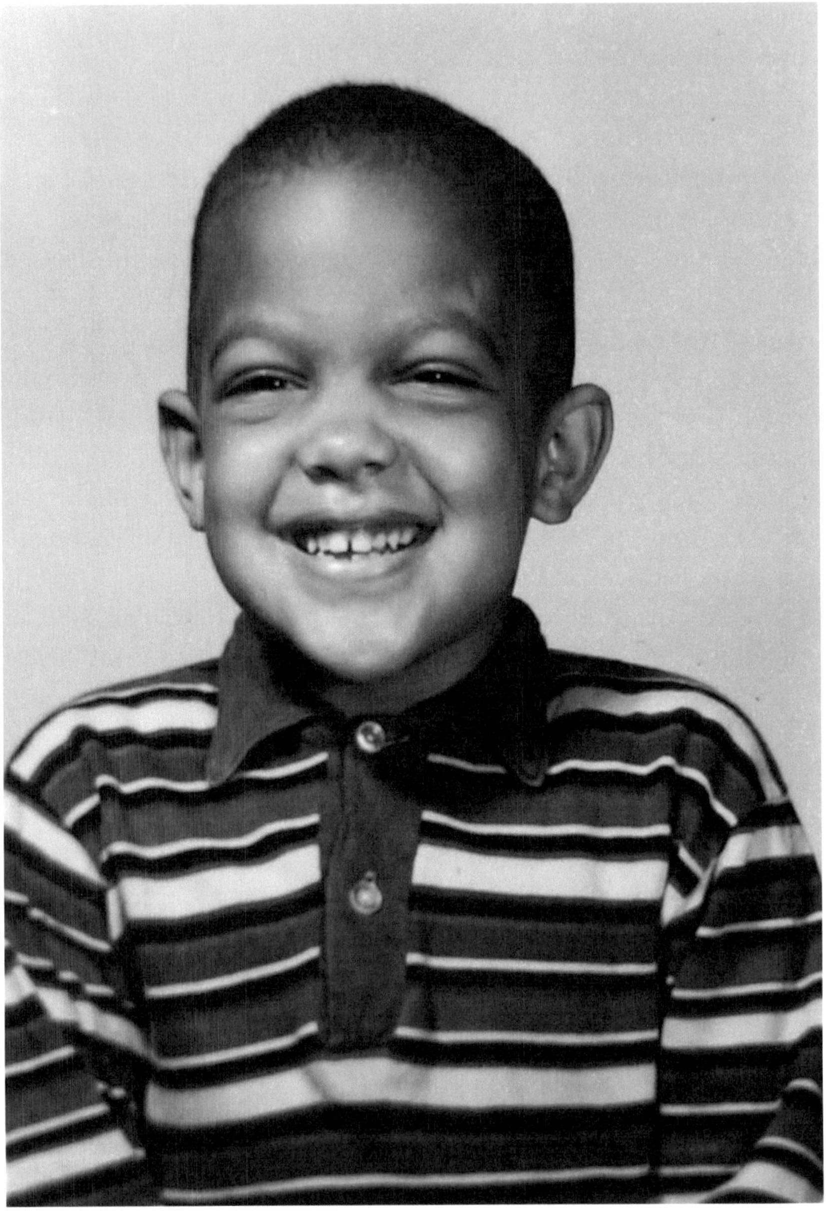

Figure 1.2. Julius "Scotty" Scott student photo when he was a first-grade student at MacGregor Elementary School, Houston, in 1961 (photograph courtesy of Ann Scott).

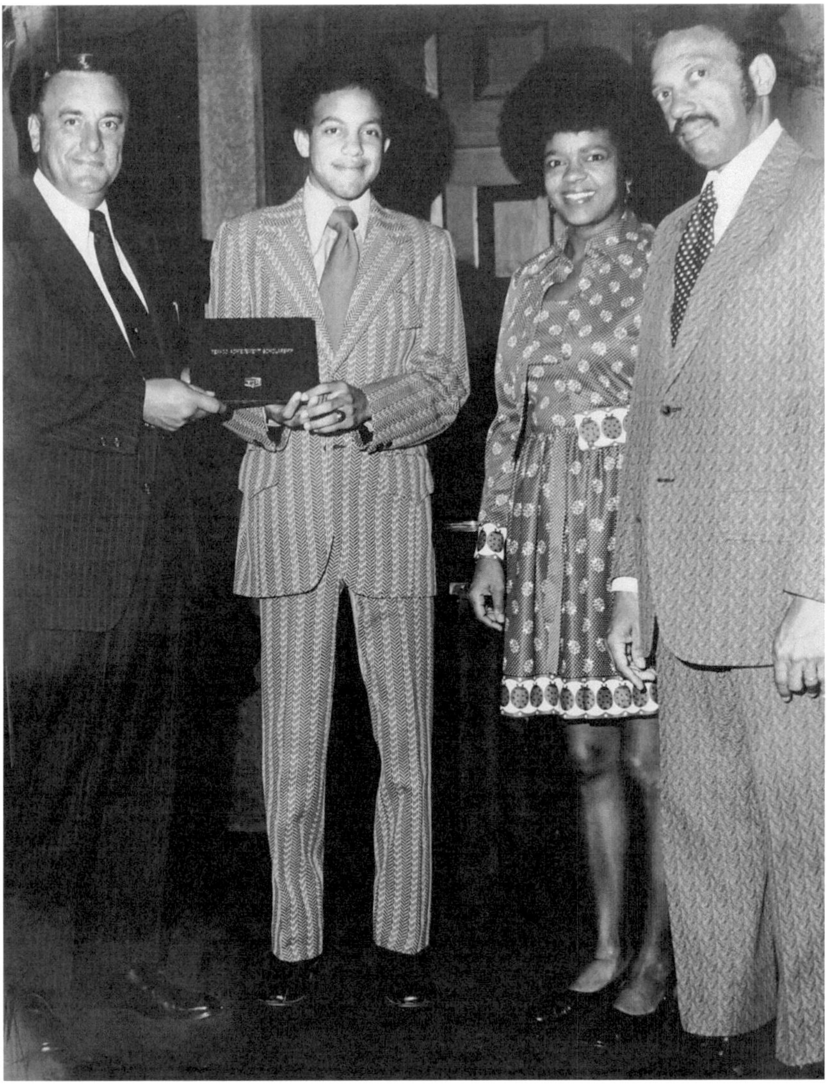

Figure 1.3. Julius with his parents, Ann and Julius Scott, Jr. (photograph courtesy of Ann Scott).

Springs, which included being named a National Merit Scholar semifinalist (Anonymous 1972) and subsequently, a National Merit Scholar Finalist (Figure 1.3).

Since he was familiar with Providence from the time when his family lived there (his father was assistant chaplain for Brown University in 1965–1966 and delivered a Baccalaureate sermon there in 1971), Julius decided to attend

Brown University beginning in the fall of 1973. After he had been diagnosed with diabetes, he was mostly careful to eat sensibly and to monitor his blood sugar. He was also an avid soccer player and bicyclist, so he was in excellent physical shape. Of course, he spent much time sitting in the library, reading books on the history of the United States, Europe, and the Caribbean.

On receiving his BA in history with honors, he began graduate school at Duke University, ironically—where he had earlier taken classes as part of the Stouffer Fellowship Program. His focus on Atlantic world history resulted in his much-acclaimed PhD dissertation and later his award-winning book, *The Common Wind*, discussed in Chapter 5. While carrying out research for his dissertation, he came across newspaper articles concerning the fate of Isaac Sasportas, a French-Jewish merchant who was executed in Jamaica, in December 1799 for his support of a slave revolt there (Scott 2018: 204). While only briefly mentioned in his dissertation, Julius followed up on this incident and presented several papers on Sasportas at conferences. A draft of this work appears in Chapter 6.

However, it was during his time at Duke when he was living in Durham, North Carolina, that he became the human for a particular dog whom he named Mogie, after the nickname of his favorite jazz trumpeter, Lee Morgan. Mogie was a medium-sized dog who appeared to be a combination of an Australian shepherd, a border collie, and a dachshund. He was mainly black with brown eyes, with tan face marking and underbelly, a long furry tail, and short legs (Figure 1.4).

Julius's close relationship with Mogie is described in Chapter 2. Mogie followed Julius everywhere—in his travels to visit his parents, who had retired in Hilton Head, South Carolina; to New York City, where he had taken up a one-year appointment as visiting associate professor of history at New York University in 1996; and to Ann Arbor, when Julius began his appointment as assistant professor at the University of Michigan in 1997.

Mogie was a very sociable dog and in many ways, he and Julius were great companions for one another. Mogie was very smart, too. For instance, when Julius would call one of his friends to arrange the meeting time for going to the Dog Club:

> Mogie got the idea that when Julius talked on the phone, that it was just before going out. So Mogie would get excited and interested when the phone rang and when Julius talked on the phone. Eventually Mogie could even assess by the

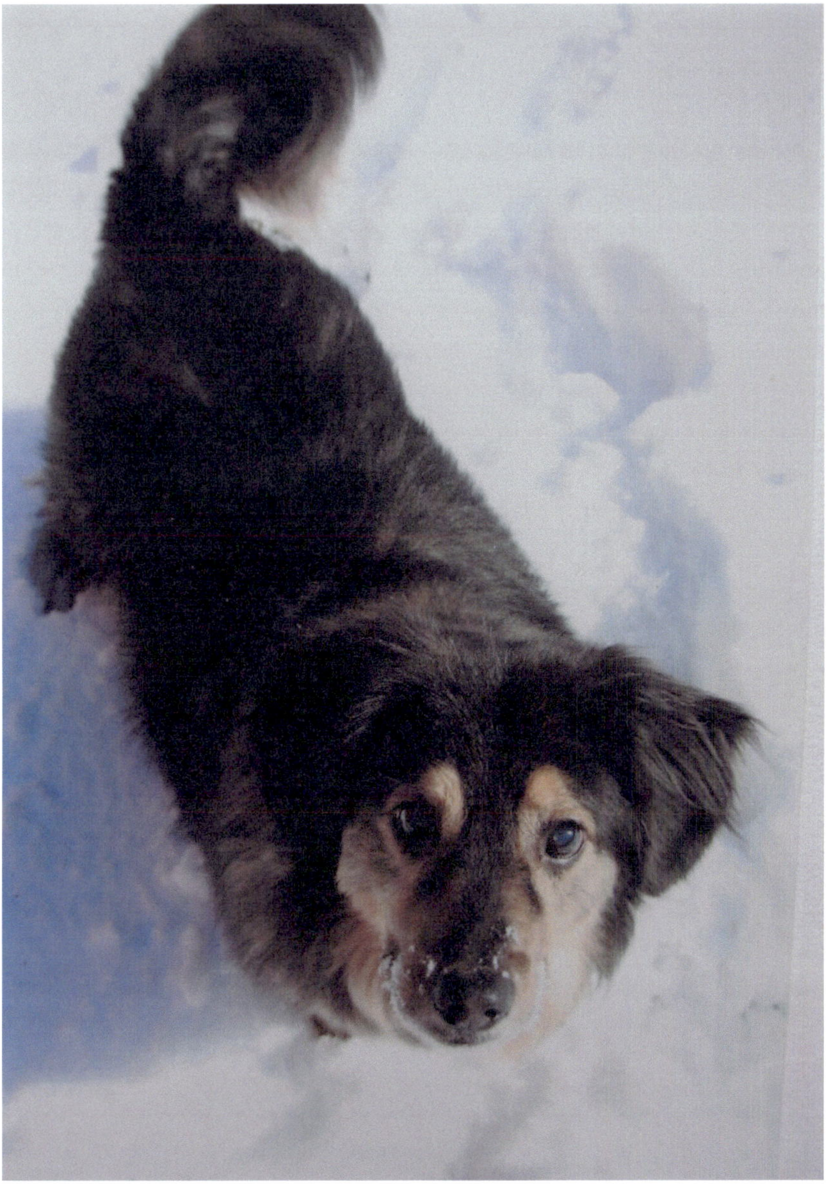

Figure 1.4. Mogie, Julius's dog, Ann Arbor, Michigan, February 2006; photograph by E.P. Renne.

conversation that it was about to end ("ok, good talking, etc.") and he would run to the door in anticipation. "This dog can understand me," Julius said.

When another friend was coming to visit and Julius was vacuuming in preparation, instead of barking at the vacuum cleaner as he usually did, Mogie went to the front door window and looked out, waiting for the expected guest to come. "This dog knows me too well, it's embarrassing and a bit frightening" (Journal, February 20, 2013).

Julius taught Mogie many tricks and took him for the "biscuit walk" at night, just before going to bed. He also teased Mogie: "Julius was playing with Mogie's toy dog [and wouldn't let him have it], which made Mogie furious and powerless at the same time" (Journal, August 16, 2008). But the magnet that Julius's father gave him, which Julius put on his refrigerator door, expressed Mogie's true position in the Scott household: "This house is owned and operated solely for the comfort & convenience of the DOG!"

Having Mogie made continuing complications from diabetes more bearable for Julius.

When he precipitously left New York for his leg amputation at the University of Michigan Hospital in 1997, he had to leave Mogie in the neighborhood kennel although his father and brother brought Mogie to Ann Arbor. Of course, Julius had to learn how to walk with a prothesis and his mother stayed with him for three months as he recovered from surgery. She walked Mogie until Julius was able to take over, wearing his prosthesis (Renne 2022. Interview: Ann Scott, November 22, 2022).

Mogie was also with Julius when he moved to his single-story house on Santa Fe Trail in Ann Arbor in December 2007. The house had two bedrooms, two bathrooms, a study, and a large living room and kitchen. He was overjoyed to be in such a spacious home with furnishings that he liked, with his stereo and many records, as well as with his collection of paintings and photographs of jazz musicians that adorned the walls. "Julius has been so happy lately, he just loves his house. It is very nice and he's kept it up" (Journal, August 6, 2009; Figure 1.5).

Having settled in Ann Arbor, Julius appreciated that teaching and seminar presentations at the University of Michigan enabled him to pursue his love of jazz. In February 2015, he gave a talk at the Department of Afroamerican and African Studies: "The Coltrane-Muhammed X session went well—and Julius was very happy. It was well-received, Julius was so good" (Journal, February 20, 2015). And in the fall of 2017, he created the course, "A Love Supreme: John Coltrane, the Sixties, and 'Jazz,'" that he taught in the Department of History, and described in the course syllabus:

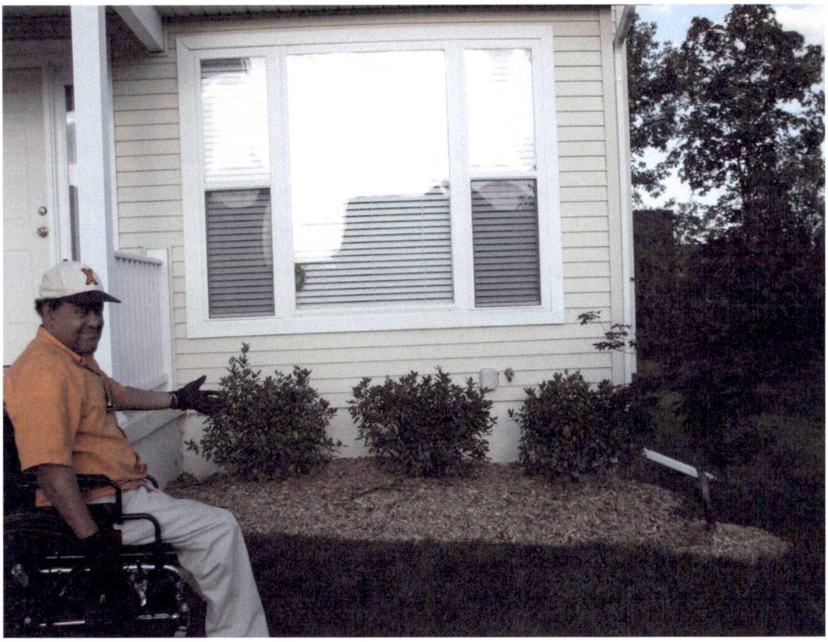

Figure 1.5. Julius proudly showing his house at 3811 Santa Fe Trail, Ann Arbor, Michigan, August 31, 2009; photograph by E.P. Renne.

> Artists contributed in important ways to the social and political developments of the "long" 1960s. This course focuses on various important roles played by jazz musicians in the period from the mid-1950s through the early 1970s, paying particular attention to the career of legendary saxophonist John W. Coltrane (1926–1967). Not only did Coltrane and figures associated with him engage in remarkable musical explorations, questioning and pushing to their limits the very boundaries of African American and Western musical expression, Coltrane's personal example came to embody what admirers—ranging from African American cultural nationalists to seekers of religious enlightenment—defined as a committed artist dedicated to values and concerns of the 1960s—social transformation, political change, and spiritual uplift, freedom (Scott 2017).

Along with talks, courses, and *The Common Wind* events, he also attended jazz performances in Chicago:

> Julius and Alex went to a jazz club, it was really good, they enjoyed it. And Julius was pleased with the various attention he's been getting. At his session, people were lining up to get their books signed. Really, it was so good that he could

> come to Chicago and see people and get all the praise for his book (Journal, January 5, 2019).

And in Detroit:

> Julius mentioned that David [his brother] is coming. And it's the weekend of the Detroit Jazz Festival so they'll have plenty to do (Journal, August 18, 2017).

Julius was especially pleased to see and hear the Wayne Shorter Quintet at the 2017 Festival (McCollum 2017), although he had low blood sugar which he fortunately managed:

> Julius said that he had low blood sugar at the Jazz Festival and he knew it when someone talking to him made no sense. So he drank two juices and David bought some food.
>
> "Did David know you had LBS?" "No, I didn't tell him" (Journal, September 7, 2017).

He did not want to worry his brother with more of his diabetic problems as David had already made an enormous effort to help Julius by donating one of his kidneys.

While the technology for providing insulin and measuring his blood sugar improved over the years, the continuing hardening of his blood vessels caused by plaque buildup from excess glucose had many detrimental consequences. Reduced circulation in his extremities led to successive surgeries of his toes, then his feet, then his lower legs, and finally the tips of his fingers. His kidneys and heart were also affected. In May 2004, he had a kidney transplant, which lasted for twelve years, after which he went to a dialysis clinic for the rest of his life. A heart attack in March 2008 led to coronary artery bypass surgery later that month.[2] The sequence of these diabetes-related incidents is discussed in Chapter 4. Yet despite the increasingly frequent surgeries, hospital stays, limited eyesight, and extreme fluctuations in his blood sugar levels, Julius managed to attend concerts, academic conferences, award ceremonies, and to visit family and friends (Figure 1.6).

---

[2] Mayo Clinic, Coronary artery bypass grafting surgery, 2022, www.mayoclinic.org/tests-procedures/coronary-bypass-surgery/about/pac-20384589.

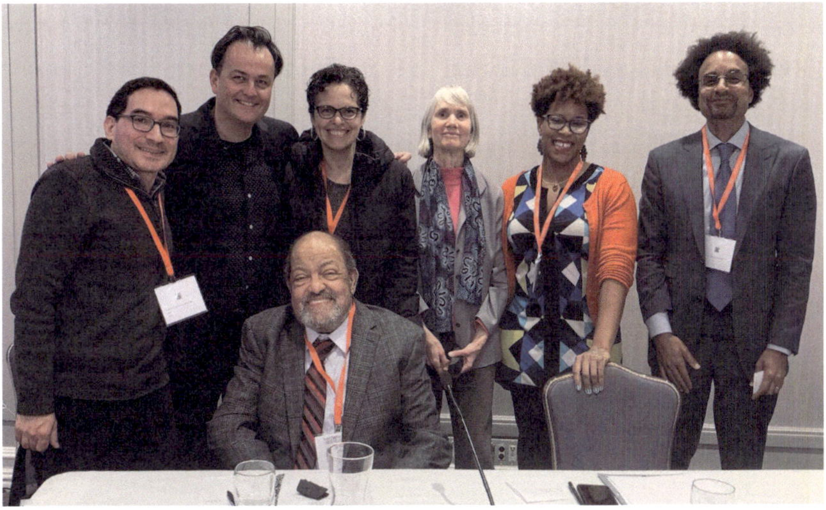

Figure 1.6. Julius attended the American History Association meeting and participated in the panel, "After The Common Wind: Atlantic Studies and the Work of Julius S. Scott III," Chicago, January 3, 2019; courtesy of Julia Gaffield.

Conclusion

Julius said that people used to call him Sherman and his father, Mr. Peabody, referring to the Bullwinkle cartoon series (Journal, December 4, 1999).[3] In it, Mr. Peabody, "the world's smartest dog," and "his boy, Sherman," would travel back in time by stepping into the WABAC [Way-Back] machine. This humorous characterization of Julius and his father was in some ways appropriate although it was Julius who went back in time to study 18th century Caribbean history. One might say that by using archival documents, library collections, 18th-century newspaper articles, as well as his discussions with his professors and colleagues, Julius used these things as his own personal Way-Back machine.

We are fortunate that his meticulous scholarship enabled us to join him. In the chapters that follow, Julius's own history and his personal qualities may more intimately be seen, from getting his very own dog, Mogie, discussed in Chapter 2 and his experience of having his very own—segregated—bathroom when he first attended MacGregor Elementary School, in Houston, Texas, examined in Chapter 3. The journal entries describing the consequences of his having type 1 diabetes and the accumulating assaults on his physical health and mental acuity provide readers with an intimate sense of the relentless

[3] Bullwinkle Studios LLC, Ward Productions, 2014.

effects of diabetes in Chapter 4. His much-acclaimed research on the myriad ways that news of the Haitian and French revolutions moved through the Caribbean world are discussed in Chapters 5 and 6. Not surprisingly, as the first Black student to integrate Southern schools, which included his first-grade class in Texas and later, secondary schools, first in Atlanta and then in Alabama, along with his family background, his experiences enabled him to astutely observe racism in its various forms, including in Ann Arbor, Michigan, which is considered in Chapter 7.

Throughout his life, Julius managed, despite his terrible illness, to carry on, with ingenuity, grace, and humor as several journal entries suggest:

> Julius was trying to photocopy something at the library, but he couldn't get his Mcard to work. He didn't have anything to write with and he couldn't read the screen to photocopy with the new Mcard, so he sat down and memorized what he needed (Journal, January 12, 2010).
>
> Julius's session at the Latin American Studies meeting went very well, his paper was well received and he had a great time. So it's good he went, it's exactly what he needed.
>
> "Well, it's too bad people liked your paper, it undermines your feelings of being marginal and incapable."
>
> "No, it doesn't."
>
> "Julius, you're impossible."
>
> "No, I'm very possible" (Journal, September 7, 2001).

And when, after the amputation of his second leg and his having to learn to walk with two prostheses, he attended a University of Michigan faculty meeting in the fall of 2009:

> He went to the History Department meeting, walking on his prostheses. People were clapping and cheering, someone even cried. And one of his colleagues at the Center for Afroamerican and African Studies said that he'd been an inspiration to others (Journal, October 22, 2009).

Although Julius didn't believe it, it was true—"People like him so much, it's just a blessing" (Journal, September 20, 2008). This idiosyncratic biography of Julius S. Scott III—"Scotty"—ends with many of the condolence memories of Julius written after his passing.

Chapter 2
My Human, Julius

Mogie was a stray dog—a puppy, actually—that Julius could not resist adopting, as he explained.

> The first time I saw Mogie, he was wandering around the Duke campus. One of the undergraduates had decided they couldn't keep him and put him in a box outside the dormitory. But Mogie jumped out of the box and escaped. It was a Friday, the day after Thanksgiving.
>
> So we took him to the local animal shelter and left him there. Then, on Monday we decided to look in on him, to see if he was ok. When we found him, he was lying in a small, caged pen on a small blanket but looked up when we walked up. I went back at the end of the week. He was in the same place but he didn't look up. I went back again on the following Monday, he was just lying there and looked so sad. Then and there, I decided to adopt him. He was too nice-looking a dog to just leave him there to die (Renne 2019a. Interview: Julius Scott, November 30, 2019).

Julius took Mogie to his apartment and got a crate where he kept him when he went out:

> I couldn't just leave him so I used the crate when I was going out. I would put Mogie in it
>
> And when I came back, I'd take him out of the crate and take him for a walk. Eventually, he got used to the crate and he would just go in the crate on his own. But that wasn't true at first, I'd have to run around to catch him and put him in the crate (Interview: Julius Scott, November 30, 2019).

According to the veterinarian who looked over Mogie, he was about three months old—still a puppy. So Julius decided to do all the things one is supposed to do when getting a new puppy. First, he gave Mogie his name:

> Somebody brought me a dog-raising book that said if you are naming a dog, you need to name it with two long vowels. Mō-giē was the nickname of my favorite jazz musician, Lee Morgan, they called him Mogie when he was alive. So it seemed like a good two-long-vowel dog name (Interview: Julius Scott, November 30, 2019).

Then, he taught Mogie some basic commands such as sit, stay, and come. He used Milk-Bone dog biscuits to reward him when he obeyed (Figure 2.1).

Julius also advised Mogie on how to behave with other animals, such as cats:

> Mogie and I went to Sue and David's house in Durham, where there were two cats. The older cat used to stay off the floor when we came over to visit. But the kitten had no sense and would walk up to Mogie and bite his ears and fearlessly taunt him. Mogie would look up to me as if to say, "Please tell me I can chase this pesky kitten." And I would say, "Now Mogie, let's show people that dogs and cats can get along." So Mogie would ignore the kitten's provocations. This behavior also encouraged the older cat, which would jump down off the counter or chair or wherever it had been hanging out and would lay down right in front of Mogie. It would stretch its body and roll over, while Mogie looked on (Journal, February 6, 2009).

Julius would provide Mogie with more fun activities. There was a park not far from campus where Julius would take Mogie for the Durham Dog Club. It was a large, fenced area where people brought their dogs and let them run around to play with other dogs. As he explained:

> There was one dog named Greta, a female dog that was owned by some good friends of mine. We used to take them for walks together so Greta and Mogie became good friends. Greta was a name he recognized. If you called the name Greta out, he would look up since he knew you were talking about Greta (Renne 2019a, Interview: Julius Scott, November 30, 2019).

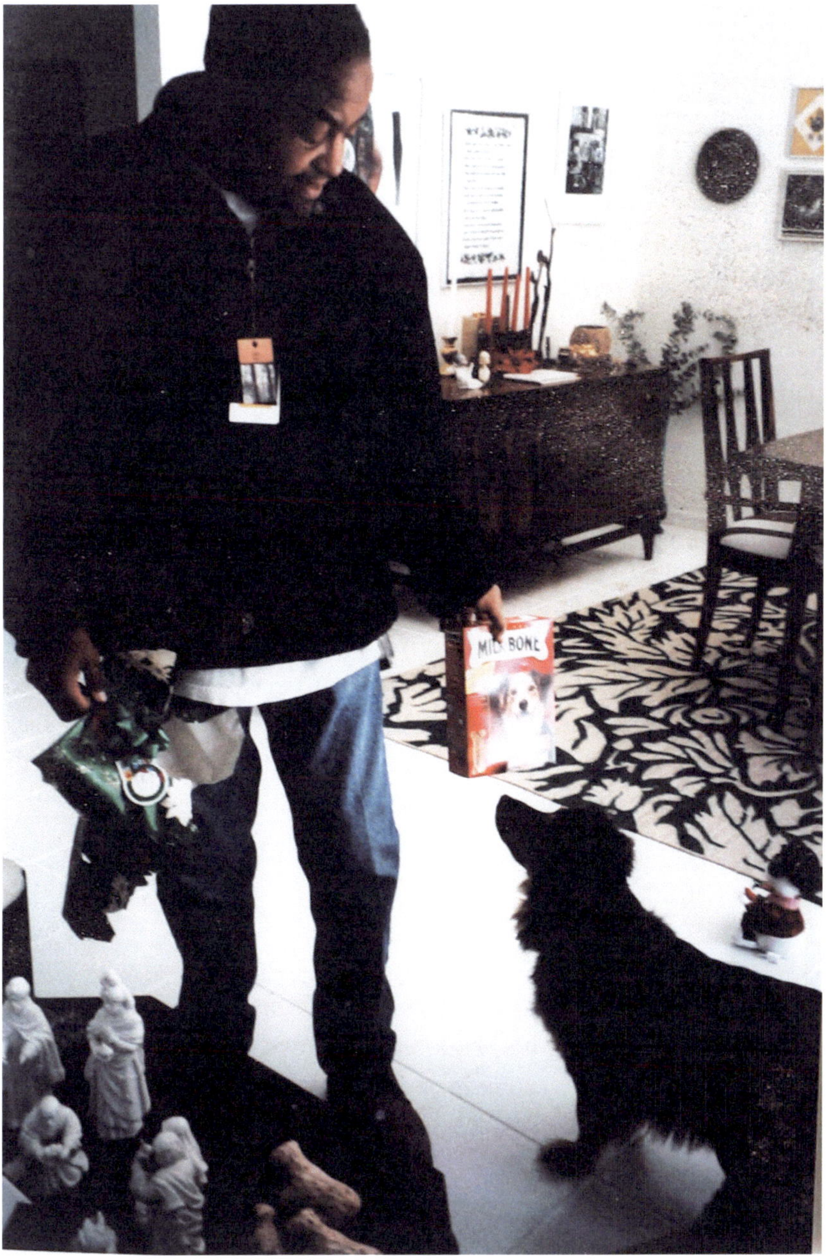

Figure 2.1. Julius showing Mogie his Christmas present, a box of Milk Bones, Hilton Head, South Carolina, December 1999; photograph courtesy of Ann Scott.

Mogie accompanied Julius when he had a visiting faculty appointment at New York University (NYU). Julius would take him for walks in Washington Square and up and down the sidewalks toward 14th Street. Mogie was a most fastidious walker and never walked on sidewalk grates.

He also had an accurate nose. For as Julius's foot became more and more infected, one day Mogie sniffed it and backed away, whimpering. It was Mogie's behavior that alarmed Julius so much that he went to the NYU Hospital where he was told that his lower leg needed surgery. He stayed in hospital for about two weeks where they administered antibiotics but did not perform surgery since Julius was scheduled to return to the University of Michigan to take up a permanent position there. So he left Mogie in a kennel and he and his mother flew to Detroit. They were immediately met by a friend of Julius's who took them directly to the emergency room from the plane. Soon after they arrived, surgeons at the University of Michigan Hospital amputated his lower leg. A few days later, when Julius was still in the hospital, his father and brother, David, drove to New York City from Ann Arbor. Both Julius and his mother cried when they left for New York. Julius was very nervous, he wanted to go with them to make sure that they brought Mogie back. But they successfully picked up Mogie from the kennel, packed Julius's belongings, and then safely drove back to Ann Arbor (Renne 2022. Interview: Ann Scott, November 22, 2022).

Mogie in Ann Arbor

At first, Julius sublet an apartment in Ann Arbor and he and Mogie soon established their routines. Julius would take Mogie for his morning walk, then he would get Mogie his breakfast of Science Diet kibble. Julius would prepare his papers for teaching, put Mogie in his crate, and leave for campus. When he got back, he took Mogie for his late afternoon walk and gave him his Science Diet dinner.

Then they might play games that often revolved around Mogie's toys or his chewy hide twists. One evening, Mogie decided he wanted to play a game with his chewy (and dog biscuits) called "Get it." He played with the chewy for a while, then left it until Julius said, "Get it!" But Mogie didn't think that all of the games that Julius came up with, like roller-ball and Oh-Oh (aka Get the Hedge-hog and Dragon) were all that great, even though he loved his hedge-hog (Journal, October 21, 2005).

One special toy that Julius's mother gave Mogie was a wind-up toy resembling James Brown, which when wound up would sing "I'm a Soul Man." Every so often Julius would say, "Mogie, I sure would like to hear 'I'm a Soul Man.'" So Mogie would run to wherever the toy was and would bring it to Julius who wound it up. Then Mogie would push it a few times until it played the song.

Another game that Mogie played was called "Attention!" Julius would say, "Attention!" and Mogie would answer, "Bark, bark." Julius later revised it to "Heil Mogie!" and Mogie would answer, "Bark!" (Journal, January 17, 2009).

Just before bedtime, Julius would take Mogie for his late-night walk, the "biscuit walk," which they both religiously observed:

> After taking Mogie out for a short late night walk, I would give Mogie three Milk-Bone dog biscuits that I would put up on the bed's back frame railing. Mogie learned how to get his biscuits, one at a time, but only when I said it was ok.
>
> So Mogie would sit and look at me, waiting in the doorway until I would say, "Ok, get one." Standing up on the bed and with his left front paw on the railing, he then took one biscuit into the hall to eat ("Go, go, go," I would say). Then he would come back, sit down, and wait until I would say, "Ok, Mogie, get another biscuit!" (Renne 2019a. Interview: Julius Scott, November 30, 2019).

Mogie Songs

Along with his games and toys, Julius made up the lyrics for many songs for Mogie that reflected TV show theme songs, such as the Dick Van Dyke Show ("My name is Mogie Dogie, I've gotta me a scrogie, and have a human who takes care of me, boop-boop…"). His most popular Mogie song, however, was called, "My Name is Mogie." It also included mention of one of Mogie's favorite squeaky toys, his hedge-hog:

> My name is Mogie, and I'm a very good dog
> My name is Mogie and I have a hedgy-hog
> Mogie's my name, hedge-hog's my game…
>
> My name is Mogie and I come when you call,
> My name is Mogie, and I'm the best of them all,
> Mogie, Mogie, hedge-hog.

Julius came up with other versions of the Mogie song. After coming back from the biscuit walk one evening, Julius sang a new Mogie song about "Strangers in the Night." He also conceived a song based on "Ring of Fire," that was sung from the hedge-hog's perspective of Mogie. It was called "Rings of Teeth": "…and they hurt, hurt, hurt those rings of teeth, those rings of teeth…" (Journal, September 23, 2003).

Julius also did an imitation of Mogie singing a Julius song. "My name is Julius, I have me a screwlious."

"What's a screwlious?" Julius asked.

"So, what's a scrogie?" Mogie asked. "When you sing, 'My name is Mogie, I have me a scrogie' " (Journal, February 25, 2005).

There were so many Mogie-related songs that one night, Julius came up with an amusing story about Mogie being tired of hearing the uncountable songs he'd made up for every TV show theme song and anything else—commercials, popular songs, opera—that he could think of. So Mogie went into the kitchen and stuffed his ears with cotton. Julius then did a perfect imitation of Mogie stuffing cotton in his ears. "And that," Julius said, "explains why Mogie's gone deaf" (Journal, October 26, 2006).

Mogie and Julius: Conversations, Dreams, Benedictions

But even if Mogie eventually lost his hearing, he and Julius carried on numerous conversations, although Julius dominated them, with Mogie being the patient listener, perhaps because he couldn't hear (Figure 2.2). For example, one night when they were watching the TV serial, NCIS (Naval Criminal Investigative Service), Julius translated the title for Mogie as "No cats in sight," which made sense to Mogie (Journal, October 30, 2006).

Another night, they had a conversation about how Mogie would care for his human. When Julius asked Mogie if he was going to take his human for walks, Julius answered, speaking for Mogie. "Yes, I would and then I'd give him his biscuits on the side of the bed. Then I would nod to Julius when it was time for him to take one, just as he does for me."

Some of their conversations were more academic. For example, when Julius was sitting on the couch in the living room, with Mogie at his feet, Julius gave a lecture on the parallel evolution of humans and dogs and how they got along together. Mogie had a bored expression on his face the whole

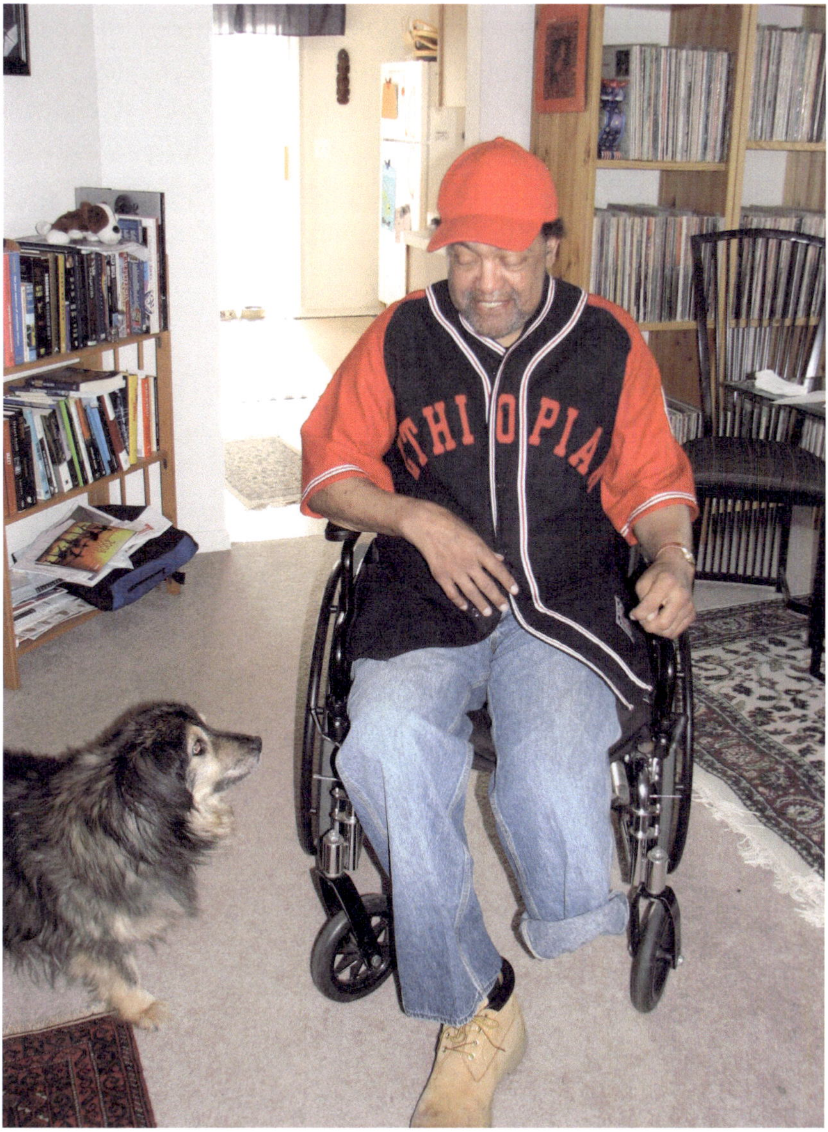

Figure 2.2. Julius and Mogie in conversation, Ann Arbor, Michigan, April 28, 2009; photograph by E.P. Renne.

time until Julius said, "go for a walk together," which sparked Mogie's interest in this historical process.

Sometimes Julius's accounts of the relations between humans and dogs were more critical as when one Sunday morning, Julius gave Mogie a short sermon on dogs' complicity with plantation owners who used them to track runaway slaves (Journal, October 19, 2003). Later, the same day, perhaps after Mogie had thought about this situation, Julius said that Mogie wanted him to know that there were dogs in ancient Egypt (Journal, November 10, 2009).

What with all their discussions about historical events, Mogie announced that he wanted tenure and that he was going to talk it up with the Dean of Dogs. "Who's that?" Julius asked. "Dean Packer," Mogie replied, referring to Packer, a dog owned by one of Julius's good friends (Journal, November 16, 2003).

Aside from these academic discussions, some of their conversations had a religious tenor. Thus, one night when they were both lying on the bed, Julius covered Mogie with the duvet. For some reason, Mogie didn't object to having his head covered like a monk's. So Julius started singing an ersatz Gregorian chant and then imitated Mogie giving a benediction: "May treats rain down upon you!" Upon hearing the word "treat," Mogie jumped off the bed and ran into the hallway, looking for his treat (Journal, April 27, 2004).

Dreams

Their worldly historical and spiritual conversations were occasionally superseded by stories of dreams that Julius had had that included Mogie. One night, Julius had a dream about some type of dog medicine that he wanted to buy for Mogie. You could tell it was working when a blue halo appeared above the dog's head. So Julius bought it and gave it to Mogie, after which he walked around with a little blue halo above his head, like a dog angel without wings (Journal, January 31, 2009).

Julius remembered another dream, one that Mogie had described to him. In it, Mogie was dreaming about being a human and how great it would be just to go into a store where there were rows and rows of chewies and stuffed animals and you could get anything you wanted just by giving the people these little bits of paper. Julius patted Mogie on the head (Journal, November 5, 2006).

"Yes, that was a very good dream," Julius said, "Unlike the dream I had last night of the 'Grim Rover,' following you around."

Sometimes one of Mogie's toys was included in their conversations. As they were sitting in the living room, watching TV, Julius said that the little hedge-hog toy was telling him naughty stories about Mogie. Another time,

Julius was explaining dialectical materialism to the hedge-hog and Mogie; Mogie would cock his head, looking as if he was intensely interested. Then Mogie would jump up and kiss Julius in order to get him to pet him.

Empathy

Along with their innumerable conversations, Mogie and his human, Julius, had many unspoken communications. Julius became more and more prone to low blood sugar episodes of varying degrees of dangerousness. They usually occurred late at night or in the very early morning. He might thrash around in bed, he might pass out, or he might fall out of the bed. The solution was usually drinking one or two boxes of fruit juice and then eating a sandwich.

Mogie often sensed when his human was having a low blood sugar episode and skulked around the bed, knowing something was wrong and trying to alert Julius to the problem.

Another time, Julius had very serious low blood sugar and fell out of bed, knocking over a glass which broke and cut his foot. Mogie was so concerned that he stayed by Julius's side, knowing something very bad had happened (Figure 2.3).

Sometimes Julius needed a glucose injection if drinking juice didn't work, and if that didn't help, the hospital would be called for emergency care. Usually this meant a few hours in the emergency room until his blood sugar level could be increased and stabilized. When Julius got back to his apartment, he went to bed. Mogie had been put in the bathroom to keep him out of the way, but when he was let out, he sniffed and sniffed, then raced into the bedroom and jumped onto the bed with Julius.

Mogie also surprised Julius late one night when he took Mogie for his late-night biscuit walk. By that time, Julius could no longer walk with a cane and got around in his wheelchair. Mogie had learned how to walk with the wheelchair but sometimes had trouble doing it, especially when his leash got tangled up with the chair's wheels. That particular night, Mogie's leash got so tangled that Julius had to get out of the chair and sit on the ground to free the leash from the wheels. He had to let Mogie off the leash to do so. When he did, Mogie took off into the pitch-black night and Julius thought to himself, "Who can I call to come help me find Mogie?" It was around midnight and it took a long time to get the leash untangled. While Julius was lying on the

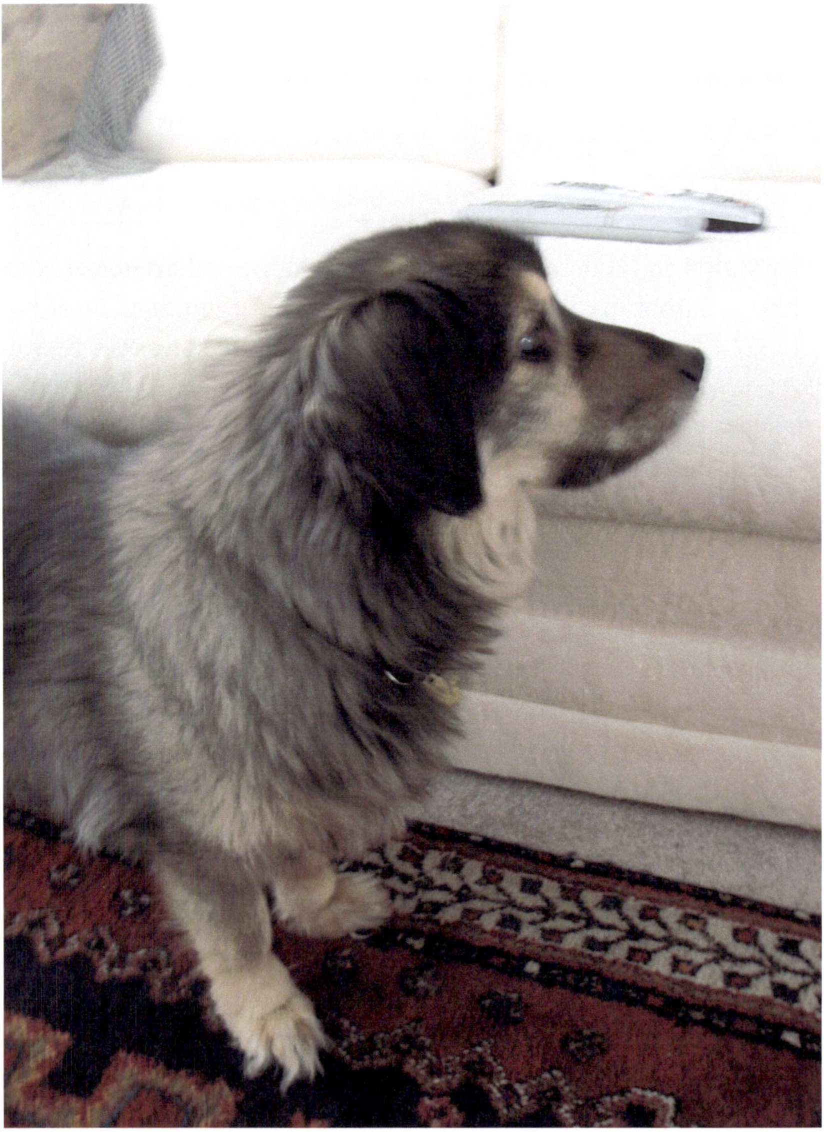

Figure 2.3. Mogie showing concern for Julius's health, Ann Arbor, Michigan, November 27, 2008; photograph by E.P. Renne.

ground working on it, somebody tapped him on the shoulder. He turned around and it was Mogie—he had come back! And then Mogie laid down as if to say, "Everything's cool, I'm fine." Julius got back in his wheelchair and, putting the leash back on Mogie, took him home (Renne 2019a. Interview: Julius Scott, November 30, 2019).

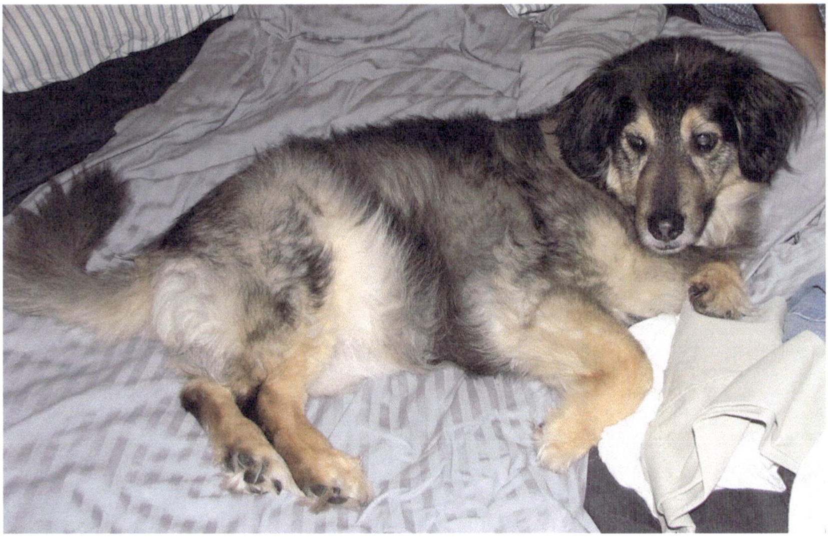

Figure 2.4. Mogie at ease, Ann Arbor, Michigan, June 6, 2007; photograph by E.P. Renne.

Julius was depressed by the difficulties of walking Mogie and continuing low blood sugar attacks, followed sometimes by equally dangerous very high blood sugar after juice and a sandwich. At times, he was certain that he was dying, a feeling reinforced by the fact that Mogie wasn't his old spunky self (Figure 2.4). In fact, Julius didn't want to take a trip to Chicago in December of 2006 because he thought Mogie was approaching his end. Although Mogie lived for another four years and Julius, for another fifteen, Julius was convinced that their lives and deaths were intertwined. Indeed, Julius said he worried about Mogie, but he also worried about himself. One night, when Mogie was sleeping on the bed with Julius, Julius woke up and sat up, whispering softly, "Mogie, Mogie," perhaps to confirm that Mogie was still alive. But by 2009, Mogie showed definite signs of his impending demise.

Mogie's Decline and Death

In September of 2009, Mogie became very sick. It seemed as though he might have had a stroke as his back legs became very weak and he could barely stand up. Although he recovered, his personality appeared to change and two months later, he behaved very badly at the groomers. As if in sympathy with

Mogie, Julius fell out of his wheelchair later that evening (Journal, November 13, 2009).

Although Mogie was alert and could still go on his evening walks, he was very fragile and wobbly. Even so, he did better walking up the street some nights than others. Also, his sight had deteriorated. It was so bad that one day, he looked at a chair with Julius's shirt on it and stood by it, thinking it was Julius.

In late July of 2010, Mogie had a crying fit and fell down in the kitchen. In August he continued to decline. One evening in mid-August, he became very restless, lying down, getting up, and crying, although he finally went to sleep halfway under the bed with his legs sticking out. A week later, Mogie had some sort of mini-stroke. He couldn't get up and when Julius stood him up, he kept falling. Julius tried to calm him down as Mogie shivered violently. He had the same scared, distant look he'd had during the crying fit in July. But then he finally was able to stand and even ate a biscuit.

"It's a reminder that Mogie's very frail and may die soon," Julius said. "He's such a sweet, sweet dog" (Journal, August 22, 2010).

Julius's concern for Mogie was also reflected in his thinking about his own health as he was thinking that he was going to die soon, too. One night, sitting on the bed and talking to himself, he said, "I want to go out with a bang." Then, the next night when he was watching the movie, *High Sierra*, he said, "I should watch it now, I may not see it again."

It wasn't clear why he felt this way, although he clearly identified with Mogie and his terminal illness. "I didn't think that I'd see Mogie alive in 2010," Julius observed, "But then I didn't think I'd be alive in 2010" (Journal, September 12, 2010).

Mogie continued to eat his food, laced with tuna fish, and to go for his biscuit walk and then get his Milk-Bone biscuits until the end of September. One morning, Julius decided that Mogie wasn't so bad off, but later that afternoon, after Mogie had thrown up, Julius realized that Mogie really was dying. The next morning, Mogie had one of his spasm attacks and his back arched up so Julius took him to the vet. Later, he gave Mogie the painkiller that the vet had given him, which helped as Mogie calmed down and went to sleep. Then Julius laid down on the bed. He just needed some down time to mourn, not just for Mogie but for the idea of Mogie, all his playfulness, affection, and all of his Mogie stories and songs.

On the 30th of September after Mogie stopped eating even his tuna fish treat and biscuits, Julius took him to the Ann Arbor Veterinarian Hospital in order to put Mogie "to sleep." The vet was very good, she gave Julius valuable support for making the decision to put Mogie down. Mogie was so miserable and out of it, his eyes were becoming sunken, he wouldn't eat, he couldn't stand up. The thing she said that really convinced Julius was that while he could give Mogie hospice care at home, like many humans, Mogie wouldn't die for some time and until then, he'd just be suffering. It was really helpful to have someone give support for the very hard decision that Julius made (Journal, September 30, 2010).

As the vet came back with the injection that put Mogie to sleep permanently, Julius placed his hands on Mogie and assured him of a better future: "Mogie, you'll be running with Greta in doggie heaven."

The vet then asked if Julius wanted to take Mogie's body back with him but he decided to have him cremated.

"Do you want the ashes?" the vet asked. "In that case, we'll have to cremate him individually."

"No, please cremate him with other dogs," Julius answered.

On getting back to the apartment, it was a very sad evening. Julius just lay on the bed, uncomfortable and crying (Journal, September 10, 2010).

"I've got to stop singing Mogie songs," he said. "But I still want to keep Mogie's food and water bowls in the kitchen."

"Anyway, I'm happy that Mogie's not suffering anymore. The night last week, when he was breathing very heavily and I woke up to find him standing next to my side of the bed, looking up at me. Or his falling down the stairs…"

****

Two months later, sitting in the bedroom one night, Julius called out, "Mogie, Mogie!" (Journal, November 17, 2010).

Chapter 3

"Thank you, God, for My Own Bathroom": Elementary School Desegregation in Houston, Texas

In the years following the 1954 US Supreme Court case known as *Brown v. Board of Education of Topeka, Kansas*, school districts in states throughout the South sought to address the ruling that instructed them to begin desegregation plans "with all deliberate speed" (Kluger 2004: 745–749). In Houston, Texas, members of the Houston Independent School District (HISD) Board of Education utilized the vagueness of this directive to hamper the implementation of the court's ruling. Thus, in January 1957, the Board determined that a study of the "integration question" would be needed to come up with an effective desegregation plan that would be acceptable to the Houston community but would also accommodate the Supreme Court directive (Kellar 1999: 96–97). However, a suit had been filed by attorneys sponsored by the Houston branch of the National Association for the Advancement of Colored People (NAACP) on December 26, 1956, which led the HISD Board to implement a plan that allowed African American students to attend previously White-segregated schools by grade. Thus, four formerly all-White primary schools in Houston began desegregation in 1960 by allowing African American children to attend first-grade classes. The following year, they were to be allowed to attend both first- and second-grade classes and so on, until all classes were fully desegregated. While the two African American community leaders, Dr. Henry E. Lee and G.W. Buchanan, who had been asked to serve on the HISD Board's Committee to Study Integration to decide on a desegregation plan, opposed this decision, a majority of the committee approved it (Kellar 1999: 97). Thus, in the fall of 1960, twelve African American six-year-old children attended elementary school classes in Houston (Kellar 1999: 137).

In the fall of 1961, Julius Scott was one of two African American children—a boy and a girl—to enter the first-grade class at MacGregor Elementary School, in south central Houston. The experiences of Julius ("Scotty") and of his parents (Figure 3.1) are examined in relation to the Houston School Board's continuing attempts to slow the implementation of school desegregation and integration in Houston. Yet as William Kellar (1999: 98) notes, there was a distinction made between desegregation and integration, which the everyday occasion of going to the bathroom at school illustrates. How Julius's parents learned about this distinctive bathroom

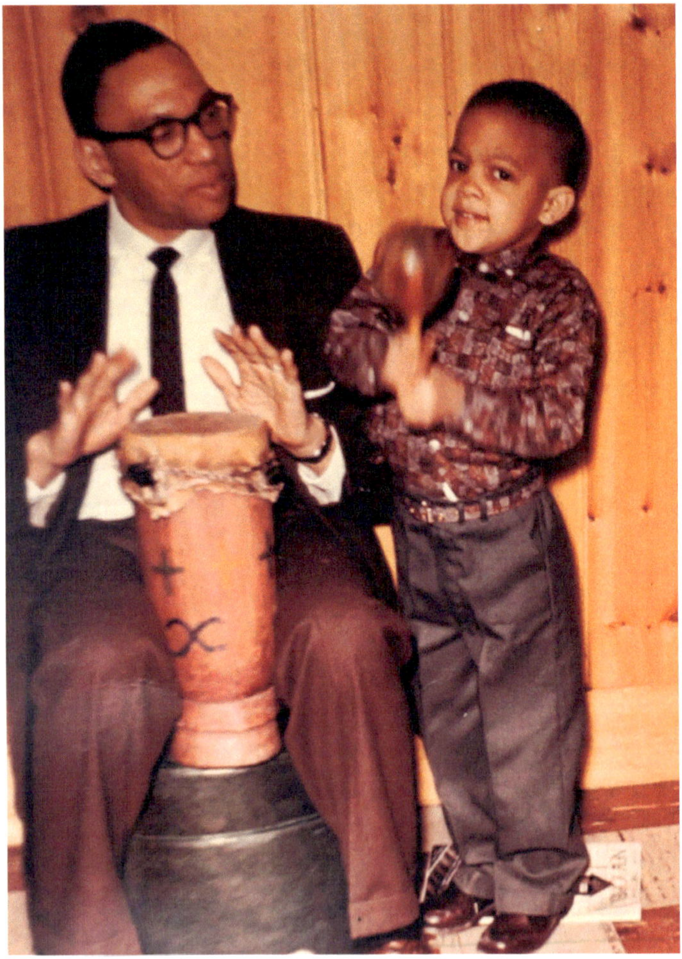

Figure 3.1. Julius S. Scott, Jr., and Julius ("Scotty") Scott III, in Houston, December 1960; photograph courtesy of Ann Scott.

practice at MacGregor Elementary and what they did about it relates to other school Board members' concerns. For in 1958, Mrs. Hattie Mae White was voted in as the first African American member of the HISD Board. The role she played in changing the Board's decisions may be seen in judgments large and small, which included her support for Julius's parents in the case of the MacGregor School bathrooms.

MacGregor Elementary School

When MacGregor Elementary School was opened in 1921, it was known as Southmore Elementary School, although in 1930 it was renamed in honor of Henry F. MacGregor, a New Hampshire-born banker and oilman who became an important civic leader in Houston. The all-White elementary school served children living in a White residential neighborhood of Houston located near the school. Julius and Jacqueline Sibley, his Black classmate, lived on Ruth Street in a Black residential neighborhood within a mile of the school. When he was in the first grade, Julius (Scotty) was taken by his grandfather, Dr. Julius S. Scott, Sr., to MacGregor Elementary School on La Branch Street. "Whoa, Scotty!" his grandfather would exclaim, as Scotty would run on ahead of him.

Although the HISD Board had made the qualifications of Black teachers an issue when discussing plans for school desegregation, all of the teachers at MacGregor were White when Julius attended. His teacher, Miss Lyda Macomb, taught reading, arithmetic, and writing to her entire class of first-grade pupils (Figure 3.2).

However, there was one practice that distinguished Julius and his Black classmate, Jacqueline, from the others. As Julius remembered it:

> Miss Macomb would announce that it was time—a couple of times during the day—for students to go use the bathroom. And she was responsible for walking with me and the Black girl, Jacqueline Sibley, and taking us outside around the back to the bathroom that they had for Black people to use. Again, mainly Black people who worked at the school [as custodians and such].
>
> So she would lead us outside around to the back and would wait for us to use the bathroom. The thing was that there was only one bathroom. It wasn't like the White students, the White students had a girls' bathroom and a boy' bathroom.

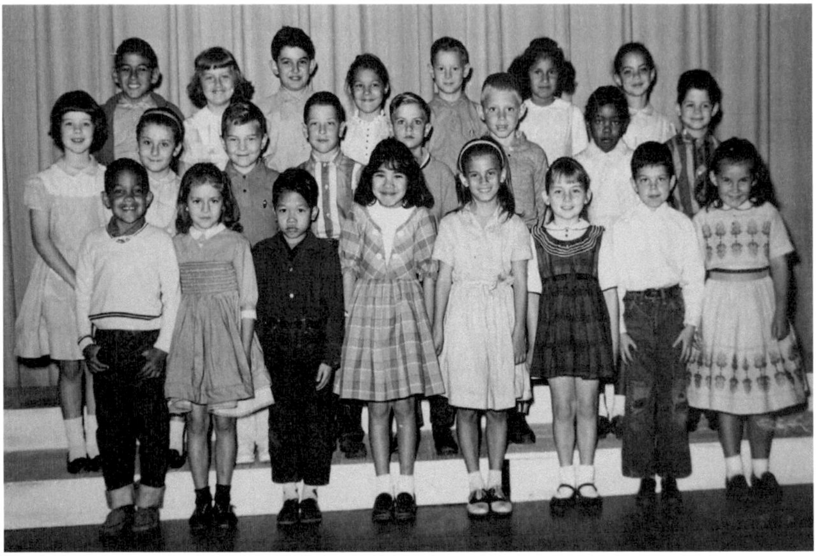

Figure 3.2. The first-grade class of MacGregor Elementary School, Houston, in 1961. "Scotty" Scott, is standing in the first row on the far left; Jacqueline Sibley is standing in the second row, second from right; photograph courtesy of Ann Scott.

> But the bathroom that was for Black people was just for one sex—everyone had to use that one. So the girl student went first and then I went second (Renne 2019b. Interview: Julius Scott, December 22, 2019).

This situation continued after the beginning of classes and neither Julius nor Jacqueline mentioned it to their parents. However, one night, when Julius was saying his prayers, his parents overheard him thanking God for something they could not understand: "Thank you God for letting me have my own bathroom at school".

> My parents didn't know anything about this and so when I said this, they asked each other, "What's he talking about?" So they asked me the next day and once they found out that I was using a separate bathroom, that the Black girl and Black boy were using a separate bathroom, they raised a fuss about it with the school board. But first they went over to MacGregor Elementary School and talked to the teacher about it. And the way they remembered it, they got a lot of hostility about their going there (Julius Scott, Interview: December 22, 2019).

When they visited the school to speak with Scotty's teacher, she made light of the practice. As Julius noted, "My mother kept remembering that my teacher,

Miss Macomb, kept saying, 'This bathroom is fine, I use it myself. There's no problem with that bathroom.'" Since Julius's parents, Julius and Ann Scott, were unable to get this bathroom practice changed through their visit to the school, they began attending meetings of the HISD Board in order to remedy the situation.

Julius's Father's Action at the Houston Independent School District Board Meeting

When Julius's parents attended a HISD Board meeting in October 1961, his father, Rev. Julius S. Scott, Jr., had hoped to question the Board about the separate bathroom practice, having spoken with Mrs. Hattie Mae (Charles) White, the one African American member of the Board.

However, the School Board members refused to hear his complaint after having asked Mrs. White if it related to desegregation. When she said that it did, the Superintendent of Houston Schools, Mr. John McFarland, said that it was an administrative matter; the Board then told Rev. Scott to put his complaint in writing.

Rev. (Dr.) Scott wrote the requested letter and again attempted to speak to the Board about the bathroom problem in a subsequent meeting. Consequently, the HISD Board members voted on a motion made by John Robinson, the Houston School Board secretary, that "the person's [Rev. Scott's] statements on desegregation be referred to the board's attorney. Robinson pointed out that a suit [*Ross v. Houston Independent School District*] concerning the board's desegregation policies has been filed against the board in federal court" (Maloney 1961); an additional issue could complicate the HISD case. While Mrs. Hattie Mae White argued that the Rev. Scott's comments "would not in any way affect the lawsuit," the Board voted (with the exception of Mrs. White) in favor of Mr. Robinson's motion.

Later, after Rev. Scott had left the meeting, he spoke with Ninian McGowen (1961), who reported the situation in the *Houston Chronicle*:

> HOUSTON—The Rev J.S. Scott, Jr. told this reporter this week that one of the things which he wanted to complain about to the Houston school board last Monday night, and one of the things to which the board would not listen, was that a Negro boy and girl in the so-called desegregated school are required to use

> the same restroom, whereas white boys and girls in the same school have a rest room for girls and a rest room for boys.
>
> HIS OWN BOY
>
> The Rev Scott said that he knew what he was talking about because his own boy attended that school and a Negro girl not a member of Rev Scott's family, have reported this condition of things at the MacGregor School, 4801 LaBranch.
>
> PREFERS PEACE
>
> The Rev Scott said that, although the school board refused the request of Mrs Charles E. [Hattie Mae] White, a board member, that he be permitted to tell his story of mixing Negro boys and girls in the rest rooms of the so-called desegregated school, he still hoped that the board would hear his story and complaint.
>
> He said that he prefers peace over litigation, but that, if the board still refuses to hear his protest against the wrong being done him and the Negro children, "I have no other recourse but to seek counsel. If it means a suit, I will have to sue."
>
> STILL SEGREGATION
>
> "My concern is to get rid of segregation in desegregated schools," the Rev Scott told this reporter. He added: "I don't want to sue anybody. I am a simple Methodist preacher concerned about humanity."
>
> Concerning the members of the school board who refused to hear his complaint, the Rev Scott said: "I will not let their discourtesy make me discourteous" (McGowen 1961).

As the head of the Wesley Foundation at Texas Southern University (one of the Historically Black Colleges and Universities, HBCU), Rev. Scott was inclined toward a peaceful settlement of the segregated bathroom matter. However, as an African American religious leader in the Houston community, he was not inclined to let the matter drop.

Consequences of Julius's Father's Intervention

It is possible that the articles published in the *Houston Chronicle*, along with pressure from Mrs. Hattie Mae White and other members of the African American community in Houston, led to a change in the bathroom policy, at least at MacGregor Elementary School. For although Rev. Scott did not file a lawsuit to change the practice of segregated bathrooms at the school, Julius and Jacqueline were allowed to go to the boys' and girls' bathrooms along with their classmates shortly after his parents' attendance at the School Board meetings.

It is also possible that the principal of MacGregor Elementary School, along with Miss Macomb, decided that it was not worth having the school involved in embarrassing legal action. Indeed, several years later, after the death of Julius's grandfather, Dr. Julius Scott, Sr., Miss Macomb told his daughter that her admiration for his accompanying his grandson to school led to her seeing school desegregation in a different—and favorable—light (Renne 2021. Interview: Ann Scott, February 5, 2021).

Julius went on to complete the first grade and continued on in the second grade at MacGregor. However, Jacqueline did not remain at MacGregor after the first grade. Indeed, in 1960 only twenty-two African American parents registered to have their children approved to attend first grade in the four elementary schools in Houston that had been selected for desegregation. Of these twenty-two child applicants, only twelve met all of the four criteria for attendance by the School Board: 1) they had to be six years old; 2) they had to enter the first grade; 3) they had to live in the district; and 4) they could not have an elder sibling attending another HISD school (Kellar 1999: 135). They were also required to have a thorough medical examination and physicians' certificate of good health along with evidence of smallpox and diphtheria immunization (Kellar 1999: 135; see also Breeden 2017: 152). Most parents did not want to subject their children to these strictures and the possible difficulties of being the first to attend all-White elementary schools. As Julius ("Scotty") explained:

> Very few Black parents wanted to send their children to first grade to face this situation. Their children were just learning what grammar school was about, they didn't need to face hostility. But my parents thought it was an acceptable thing—to participate in desegregation, although they had to be certain that everything was ok with it. So, if they thought I was having problems, they wanted to make sure that these things—such as segregated bathrooms—were taken care of. The main problem that I remember was the separate bathroom policy (Renne 2019b. Interview: Julius Scott, December 22, 2019).

Alternately, the Houston School Board officials implemented the policy of segregated bathrooms at MacGregor Elementary School as one way of placating the concerns of White parents, who worried about their children associating with Black students. As Jane Hill (2008: 21) notes, "The arrangement of racial categories within a hierarchy...produces what I will call, 'White virtue,' the idea that Whites are highest in the hierarchy because their qualities deserve this arrangement." White students deserved their own separate gendered bathrooms within the main building of MacGregor Elementary School, reflecting their supposed healthier and hygienic position in the Houston race-based social hierarchy. Black students, while having been required to have a medical examination and a physician's certificate of good health before being accepted for classes, were relegated to a single bathroom at the back of the school building as if color and contagion were synonymous.

Desegregation, White Flight, and Magnet Schools

> After the 1954 Supreme Court decision, basically what was happening in public schools in Houston was that school board members were trying to figure out ways they could limit integration but still have it be legal, to be seen as following the desegregation law. But every school system had different things that they did to make sure they limited integration and also made schools acceptable for White students. In Houston they tried to have grade by grade integration and segregated bathrooms (Renne 2019b. Interview: Julius Scott, December 22, 2019).

Thus, while the HISD Board did follow the Supreme Court's ruling to a certain degree, it attempted to obstruct the demands of African American families, such as the parents of Delores Ross and Beneva Williams, that their children be allowed to attend nearby neighborhood schools that happened to be all-White schools (Bryant 2004). In their suit, *Ross v. Houston Independent School District*, filed in federal district court on December 26, 1956, with the assistance of NAACP lawyers, the plaintiffs asked for "a definitive ruling on their legal rights;" for "the court to declare unconstitutional...[Texas] laws that mandated racially segregated public schools in Texas;" "for a permanent injunction against HISD board members from requiring segregation of public schools," and for the "HISD pay all court costs involved in this lawsuit" (Kellar 1999: 90). It was only in 1984 that the suit was handled in an out-of-court settlement (*Ross et al. v. Houston Independent School District et al.*, 1983). Yet while the public schools within the HISD have been desegregated, White flight to the suburbs in surrounding districts ("residential segregation") has led to schools within Houston with largely Black and Hispanic student populations (Breeden 2017: 382).

One solution to this problem was the implementation of magnet schools. Initially, magnet schools, which focused on special educational programs, were established to provide more racial balance within Houston district schools with predominantly Black and Hispanic students by attracting suburban White students. However, the distance from their homes, even with free busing provided by the HISD, discouraged many suburban White students—however interested—from attending. Nonetheless, Houston magnet schools continue to offer exceptional educational opportunities to students within the district. Indeed, MacGregor Elementary School is now a music magnet school, with an African American principal and predominantly African American students (MacGregor Elementary School website).

Julius "Scotty" Scott, however, did not attend MacGregor Elementary beyond the second grade. For in 1963, his family moved to Providence, Rhode Island, where his father took up a position as assistant chaplain at Brown University. In Providence, Scotty attended John Howland Elementary School, an integrated school where the majority of his classmates were White, although he remembers that there were a few African American students in his class (Figure 3.3).

Conclusion

As Weldon H. Berry, the lead NAACP attorney in the *Ross v. HISD* desegregation case, observed regarding the Supreme Court ruling of *Brown v. Board of Education of Topeka*, "It isn't a completely failed experiment, but it hasn't by any means, accomplished everything we wanted it to. Our expectations were too great. You can't legislate love" (Kellar 1999: 174). Indeed, some point to the de facto school segregation that has emerged, with public school attendance based on residence in districts with different economic means, as a consequence of the 1954 Supreme Court ruling.

Yet while this ruling was hardly a perfect attempt to address racial discrimination and socioeconomic disparities, it was a step toward racial

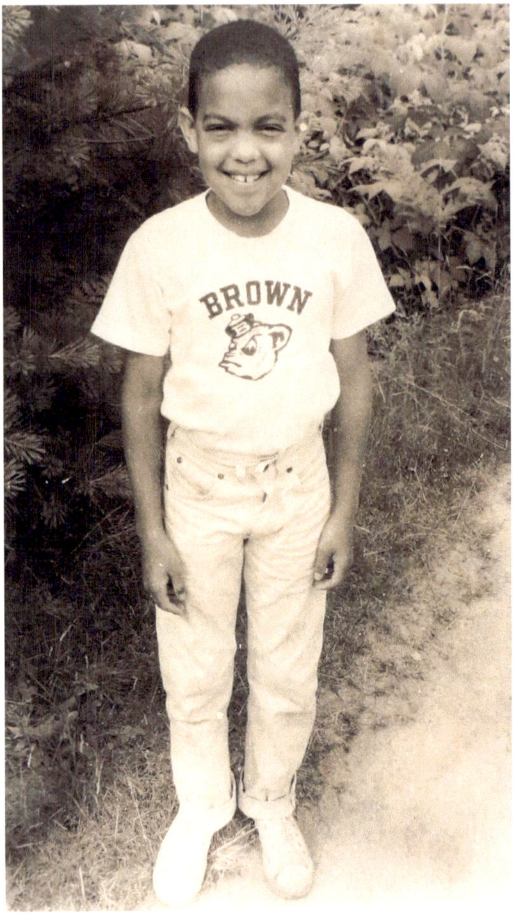

Figure 3.3. Julius "Scotty" Scott III, a student at John Howland Elementary School, Providence, Rhode Island, wearing a T-shirt from Brown University, where his father was assistant chaplain. Julius later attended Brown University and graduated *magna cum laude* in 1977; photograph courtesy of Ann Scott.

integration in Houston. This project of asserting equal rights for all continues to this day, even in the face of continuing assertions of "White virtue—that Whites are highest in the hierarchy because their qualities deserve this arrangement" (Hill 2008: 21). Yet the widespread efforts of political leaders to register African American voters and the activities of supporters of Black Lives Matter to implement police reform suggest the eventual dismantling of this hierarchy. And even the very small step of contesting the segregated bathroom policy at MacGregor Elementary School in 1961 has implemented a change in the right direction, however difficult this step might be.

Chapter 4
Diabetes: The Dangerous Disease

The disease known as *diabetes mellitus* is caused by the failure of the pancreas to produce insulin that enables cells to access glucose circulating in the blood.[1] Julius first experienced a serious diabetic event when he was 18 years old, as a freshman at Brown University. He had passed out and was taken to the hospital when his low blood sugar numbers led to the diagnosis of diabetes. He knew members of both sides of his family who were living with diabetes or had died from diabetes so that it was suspected that he had type 1 diabetes. This autoimmune condition was also attributed to his heredity since he was very active sports-wise and was not overweight.

> Julius said that he wasn't really surprised when he was diagnosed with diabetes, after he'd been horrified at what his Aunty Bess had gone through. She had told him that it was caused by eating too many sweet things so after that, he had pangs of guilt and fear that he would get diabetes (Journal, February 5, 2012).

Sometimes referred to as juvenile or type 1 diabetes, individuals with this disease needed to take insulin for the rest of their lives (Matthews et al. 2008).

Yet from the time when he was diagnosed as diabetic in 1973, there were significant changes in the delivery of insulin. When he was first diagnosed with diabetes, the main way of testing blood sugar levels was through finger sticks for blood that was measured with a glucometer, preferably four times a day. And before a meal, he would assess the carbohydrates he was eating and take the amount of insulin needed to keep his blood sugar within prescribed levels. These procedures were tedious, often inconvenient, and easier said than done. One aspect of type 1 diabetes is rapid changes in blood

---

[1] Type 1 diabetes develops when the immune system mistakenly attacks and destroys cells in the pancreas, which produces insulin (Mayo Clinic 2023).

sugar levels—so that Julius would have normal blood sugar levels and almost immediately, experience very high or very low blood sugar. For example, one day, "Julius had a low blood sugar attack at school around 11 a.m., although he was in his office at 10 a.m. and was fine. It really came down fast" (Journal, April 25, 2015). And one evening:

> Julius had a low blood sugar episode around 6:15 p.m. It came on so suddenly, he was drowsy and watching the golf game on and off. Then his mouth became distorted so he drank a juice but by that time, it was too late. His blood sugar was 40, so he was given a Glucagon injection since he couldn't drink anything else. It took about 10 minutes for him to get back; afterwards he had terrible shivers. He's ok now but is breathing heavily. It's so difficult for him, that these blood sugar drops come so suddenly (Journal, September 22, 2012).

Low blood sugar episodes could also cause incoherency and loss of balance:

> Julius got up to go to the kitchen and fell down—he had really low blood sugar, his blood sugar—it was 29. So he said, "That can't be right," and he took it again. It was 30! He's not supposed to be able to function at all with it that low (Journal, October 15, 2004).

As one of his doctors observed: "Type 1 diabetics are very sensitive to insulin." Thus, the need to drink juice and eat or to take more or less insulin had to be assessed continually.

The individual syringe and insulin vial were eventually replaced by an insulin pen, a larger syringe that was preloaded with insulin. One only had to dial the dose of insulin needed, twist on a new, small needle, and inject. However, it was the introduction of an insulin pump that enabled Julius to inject the required amounts of insulin through a thin plastic tube put under the skin on his stomach. The pump itself had both basal (short-acting) and rapid-acting (bolus) amounts of insulin so that Julius could adjust his blood sugar accordingly. However, he still needed to use a glucometer to measure his blood sugar levels, especially when he sensed that his blood sugar was getting low.

Fortunately, meters were soon developed that included continuous glucose monitoring (CGM) that could give blood glucose readings on his phone and could automatically dispense appropriate amounts of insulin from the associated pump. Julius began using a G6 CGM in December 2015 and could see his blood sugar levels on his iPhone, while also hearing beeps when his blood sugar went below 70 (low blood sugar) or above 180 (high blood sugar). While this system was easier than taking blood sugar readings four times a day, there were also problems, especially as his eyesight worsened. And with surgeries—on his right hand in 2014 and 2015 and when he lost fingers in 2017, it became more difficult to hold the pump and to manipulate the keyboard.

> Julius was much better last night even joking around about getting his fingers and arm to move. But his hand is bothering him, so surgery is pending. Dr. H. described the bone as "moth-eaten" around the large knuckle in the hand. So that bone will be cut out, back to lower in the hand where the bone was still good. They will be doing lab tests to identify the particular bacteria wreaking this havoc. Dr. H. insisted that they are a long way off from advising removal of the entire hand (Journal, December 12, 2014).
>
> Julius's surgery should be over by now, it's not clear if they are removing the middle finger or not—the nail came off the other day (Journal, May 22, 2015).

At times, he would give himself too much or too little insulin:

> Julius had low blood sugar this evening. He's been taking too much insulin for dinners with few carbohydrates. He was just sitting "watching" TV with a glazed expression. Taking his blood sugar, it was 37, which is very low (Journal, January 13, 2014).

Furthermore, the glucose monitor would sometimes give false readings, especially when blood contaminated the sensor. He would then need to find a place on his stomach or side to insert the sensor where there wasn't a chance of bleeding. And sometimes, there were problems with his insulin pump:

> Julius's pump stopped working very early this morning, He called the hospital around 9 a.m. and they were very good about connecting him, so he was able to get his Lantus insulin and syringes (Journal, April 23, 2016).

A week later, he received a new pump and his "roller coaster blood sugars" were reduced.

Progressive Problems

While technology for providing insulin and measuring his blood sugar improved over the years, the continuing hardening of his blood vessels caused by plaque buildup from excess glucose had many detrimental consequences. One of Julius's doctors said that he was helping three other African American men—all with diabetes and losing their bodies bit by bit (Journal, November 9, 2007).

Feet, Legs, and Mobility

Although Julius suffered low blood sugar incidents and problems with pain in his feet since his initial diagnosis, it was in June 1997 that the lower part of his left leg was amputated at the University of Michigan Hospital. After moving to Ann Arbor to teach at the University of Michigan in the fall of 1997, he had many medical appointments, hospitals stays, and experienced a series of amputations of parts of his feet:

> Julius looked terrible this morning, he's got another infection in his foot (Journal, February 1, 2005).
>
> Julius seemed much better last night although Wednesday night, he went to the UM Emergency Room about his toe, which was black and looked horrible; he also had a temperature (Journal, February 5, 2005).
>
> Julius is so unhappy, he said that he'll have to stay in the hospital for a few more days as his leg is discolored from the foot up to about halfway of his lower leg (Journal, February 7, 2005).
>
> Julius was good this morning, although he has a serious wound from the foot surgery (Journal, February 12, 2005).
>
> Julius's doctors said that his foot was healing very slowly, what's troubling is that the heel has cracked and the big toe is getting a sore. Julius thinks it's a matter of time, probably not long, before they'll take the foot (Journal, March 23, 2005).
>
> Julius is worried about his foot, it smelled awful yesterday and was very swollen (Journal, January 19, 2006).
>
> Julius is back in the hospital and it looks like more surgery. He's so upset. He may go along with the surgery but now he's against it and may ask that they just take the leg (Journal, February 5, 2006).

> Julius went into the hospital on Friday, July 14, 2006. The toe must have looked pretty bad, they still haven't operated, it will be tomorrow or Tuesday (Journal, July 16, 2006).
>
> The toes went, so now he's toe-less. But he seems happy and is even going to a baseball game on Sunday (Journal, July 18, 2006).

The problem with his right foot continued in the following year, although his doctors attempted to strengthen arteries and veins in his leg in early November 2007 in order to improve the circulation of blood in his leg and foot.

However, this attempt was unsuccessful so that on the last day of December in 2007, he was in the hospital as they made preparations for the amputation of his foot:

> Julius had his foot amputated on Tuesday morning, January 1, 2008. The team was good so it seemed to go well. His leg actually looks ok, swollen but not terribly so (Journal, January 3, 2008).
>
> Julius looked very good today, now that the foot is off. He saw his nurse from before his operation and showed her where the foot she'd helped him care for used to be (Journal, January 5, 2008).

The foot surgery in early 2008 was soon followed by another major surgery, that of the amputation of his lower right leg at the University of Michigan Hospital, on March 26, 2009. While the surgery wound of his leg took some time to heal, he was able to get a second prosthesis fitted so that he could walk. Nonetheless, he was still unhappy about this loss for several years after the surgery and even with his prostheses:

> When Julius woke up one morning, he was asked what he wanted for breakfast. So he asked in turn, "Do you know what I want?" "What?" "Legs," he replied (Journal, December 23, 2013).

Loss of Kidney Function

The poor circulation of blood to his kidneys had impeded their functioning, so Julius's doctors recommended that he begin peritoneal dialysis in order to remove waste products from his blood. A bag of cleansing dialysis fluid was hung from a stand, which allowed the fluid to flow through a catheter that was inserted into his abdomen. The fluid interacted with the lining of his abdomen (the peritoneum) which filtered the blood waste. The waste fluid from his abdomen then flowed through a drain line into a sterile collection bag and its contents were flushed down the toilet.

Julius began peritoneal dialysis in December 2001 although he had some problems with his catheter:

> Julius was having trouble with dialysis again this morning. They think that the catheter may have shifted. It's just one thing after another with this peritoneal dialysis. Dr. M. wasn't joking when he told Julius that the medical system had failed him (Journal, December 26, 2001).
>
> Julius feels awful, this dialysis business is just terrible, a full-time occupation (Journal, December 16, 2001).
>
> The dialysis business is scary. It seems inevitable to me that he'll get an infection. He's careful but it is so impossible to remember everything all the time. And he's having trouble seeing so when a bag leaks, he might not notice. He did look better today, even if he said he doesn't feel better (Journal, December 22, 2001).
>
> Julius had trouble draining this morning, it's a real Rube Goldberg set-up, putting liquid from a plastic bag into one's peritoneal cavity and then draining it out. It's likely that there will be complications (Journal, December 24, 2001).

Of course, there were complications. In late March, "Julius didn't drain this afternoon as there wasn't time" (Journal, March 26, 2002). The next day, he became very sick with peritonitis (when the thin layer of tissue inside his abdomen—the peritoneum—became infected) and he had to spend all night in the emergency room. It probably was the missing drain that led to this" (Journal, April 1, 2002).

So Julius was pleased when his doctors told him that they were going to start him on the Cycler, a desk-top machine, used for peritoneal dialysis (Journal, May 14, 2002). A bag with dialysis fluid was laid on top of the machine and fluid pumped into Julius's abdomen, while he lay in bed. That way, he could sleep as fresh dialysis solution automatically flowed into his abdomen and this waste fluid from his abdomen was then pumped into a sterile collection bag; later, its contents then were discarded. However, this process needed to be repeated 3–4 times during the night.

Yet it wasn't easy getting everything prepared for the Cycler, finding the correct bag of fluid, attaching the bag to the catheter, getting comfortable in bed, and starting the machine.

> Julius cried this morning, he wouldn't say why… But he was uncomfortable with the Cycler last night (Journal, June 2, 2002).

Seven months later he became ill which he attributed to the discomfort of his Cycler:

> Julius is better. Dr. M. figured out the problem of the wounding catheter that was pinching his colon, which explained the symptoms—the terrible pain and the terrible nausea and vomiting. It was interesting that the first doctor admitted that he didn't have a clue what the problem was (but at least he eliminated the peritonitis problem) and the second one stubbornly ignored the right diagnosis. He's still not out of the woods but he was much better (Journal, January 18, 2003).

The following week, Julius was told that he would need to return to the hospital in order for the catheter to be properly placed.

These difficulties with peritoneal dialysis encouraged Julius to consider getting a kidney transplant. Fortunately, his brother, David, was willing to go through all the tests and paperwork to prepare for the transplant. So, in late September 2003, Julius had some very good news. The kidney transplant was scheduled for late November or early December. However, it was only in March 2004 that his brother learned that he had passed all his tests and that they were scheduling surgery for late March or early April. Actually, the surgery finally took place on May 7, 2004:

> Post operation—they both made it with flying colors and Julius is his cranky funny self with "beautiful eyes" as one of the nurse's aides put it. It was terrifying when they were holding him downstairs and not bringing him up from "recovery" until 6 p.m. He could be seen on the gurney, all still, but when they asked him about the pain level, he said "2". He was conscious and

> even with it. Everyone greeted him, it was such a relief to see him moving, talking, and feeling ok—and making urine (Journal, May 7, 2004).

Julius did very well with his new kidney and his nephology doctor said to him ten years later, in 2014, "Five more years I hope."

Unfortunately, during a trip to Martha's Vineyard to visit with friends in 2015, he experienced extremely high blood sugar, over 600. He passed out and was taken to Martha's Vineyard Hospital where he suffered a cardiac arrest:

> They've taken Julius to the hospital, it sounds very serious. His kidney isn't doing well and he is having trouble breathing. His brother said that his heart stopped beating for a minute and that he also vomited blood (Journal, August 7, 2015).

He was then flown by helicopter to Massachusetts General Hospital (MGH) where the Intensive Care Unit (ICU) facilities for such a serious case were available. When he got there, he was unconscious. And they put him on dialysis, as his donated kidney had stopped working.

Julius stayed in MGH for sixteen days. It wasn't easy getting permission for him to fly to Ann Arbor so he could go to the University of Michigan Hospital where he was more comfortable. One of the MGH doctors gave Julius a hard time about leaving:

> He went on and on about finding the source of the infection—that could flare up during the flight—which could be delayed or longer than expected. This man also had the nerve to come in on Friday morning and wished Julius a safe flight, after trying to sabotage his discharge (Journal, August 21, 2015).

When he left the next day, a paper had to be signed saying that Julius had left Massachusetts General Hospital "against medical advice." But Julius was very glad to leave Boston:

> He was so happy when he got in his brother's friend's car, he just smiled and smiled. He did very well with conversation and was still smiling in the airport and when he got on the plane... There was no problem getting him into his seat or into the wheelchair. Seeing Julius's mood change on leaving the hospital, it was the right decision.

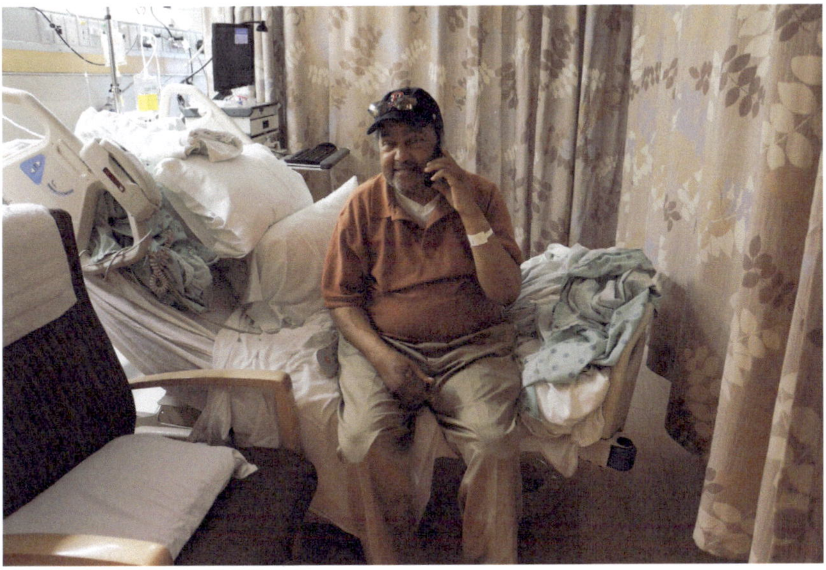

Figure 4.1. Julius was very happy to be back in Ann Arbor at the University of Michigan Hospital after leaving the Massachusetts General Hospital, even if it meant going to a local dialysis clinic on his return, Ann Arbor, Michigan, August 22, 2015; photograph by E.P. Renne.

> Julius made it without trouble to University of Michigan Hospital and Julius is much, much happier. He was confused when we'd gone (to the UM Cardiovascular Center Garden) and thought he was in another hospital. So, he's still not completely with us. But he's getting there and at least he's sleeping so he'll be able to recover. And the food is much better, his meal tonight looks appetizing and he was eating (Journal, August 23, 2015; Figure 4.1).

A week later, Julius was back home in his house in Ann Arbor. While he still had problems controlling his blood sugar, the immediate problem was the loss of his donated kidney and the need to attend a clinic for dialysis.

Rather than attempt a return to peritoneal dialysis, Julius's doctor told him that he should begin hemodialysis, when his blood would be removed from his body through a catheter, filtered through a dialysis machine, and then returned to the body as filtered blood. So he began attending the DaVita clinic in Ann Arbor, three times a week. He continued with this regimen until the end of his life.

Heart Problems

The continuing buildup of plaque on arteries and veins also affected Julius's heart, another consequence of diabetes that significantly affected his life. Following his foot surgery in January 2008, he began to suffer from intermittent chest pains. In March 2008, he experienced a minor heart attack that led to two weeks of hospitalization and surgery once again at the University of Michigan Hospital.

> A group of surgeons came in and explained his options—that he'd probably have to have surgery for the main arterial blockage in his heart, then stents for the rest (Journal, March 14, 2008).

The next day, they made preparations for coronary artery bypass surgery, referred to colloquially as a CABG.

On March 17, 2008, Julius went for his surgery, which lasted for four and a half hours. But he made it through surgery and his doctor said that he had done well. Nonetheless, the days following his surgery were not easy:

> Julius had a hard night, vomiting. He's sleeping now, he said it was painful, vomiting and that he can't talk much (Journal, March 18, 2008).
>
> Julius was feeling down but he was much better this evening, after they'd removed the chest tubes (Journal, March 30, 2008).
>
> Julius was ok this morning, but he was worried about the pain in his chest, thinking it was his heart. But the doctors assured him it was from pulling his thoracic cavity open, another reason for the term CABG (cabbage) surgery. But they later told him that he had "heart flutter" (Journal, March 21, 2008).
>
> Julius was ok last night although he coughed and was in terrible pain (Journal, March 23, 2008).

After three days, he had recovered sufficiently to be sent to a therapy center where he was supposed to be cared for until he could go home. Unfortunately, the therapy center care was insufficient and he was sent back to the University of Michigan Hospital.

> Julius had some awful news today, that the sternum bone may be infected, that there will be a series of surgeries. But they also told him that he had 2 negative blood cultures in a row, suggesting a counterindication. And Dr. K. came in

> later, after the plastic surgery crew had come in, to say that he had indeed two negative blood cultures (Journal, April 9, 2008).

After being in the hospital for another seven days, it was determined that he did indeed have an infection and he was back in surgery:

> Julius is in surgery. One of the doctors went on about some study they were preparing for publication about how before there was a 50% mortality rate with this procedure but now it's down to a small percentage. Julius started crying when he was told how everyone loved him and was praying for him (Journal, April 16, 2008).

After four days in the hospital:

> Julius had a terrible evening—he cried several times, it's so terrible. Plus the weekend night staff is especially awful and he can't stand the nurse who asked about bowel movements and then didn't help him get on a toilet seat. They couldn't figure out how to move him, the lift person was useless, and the tech person abandoned him in the bathroom.
>
> But the real problem now is that his chest skin burn isn't healing, they put some cream on it but he was in terrible pain all morning. At least they took him off the drip but now his blood sugar is very high and they won't give him enough insulin to bring it down. He really is unhappy and miserable (Journal, April 20, 2008).

But two days later, the sore on Julius's chest was finally healing and he was sent back to the therapy center. But once there, the chest wound was "draining" again. As he put it, "Déjà vu all over again" (Journal, May 12, 2008). Nonetheless:

> Julius is feeling much better, it was wonderful although he doesn't know about the continuing drainage. He seemed in a good mood, not morose or depressed, and he was joking around, "Sick people have no rights!" (Journal, May 12, 2008).

"Julius is recovering and the wound really looks like it is healing" (Journal, May 15, 2008).

He was still returned to the University of Michigan Hospital for final exams on May 25, 2008. After some confusion over his lab test results, Julius finally was discharged from the hospital and was able to return home on May 29, 2008.

He was very happy to be back home and when he went for a final meeting with his cardiologist after being discharged from the UM Cardiovascular Center:

> He made Dr. P. laugh when he said he'd have one less doctor of the forty doctors he was seeing. Dr. P. said that Julius looked good, that everything seemed to be fine (Journal, June 1, 2008).

Unfortunately, he spoke too soon as a month later in early July 2008, his chest pain returned. It was determined that while it was not caused by a heart attack, it was from an infection of his sternum:

> Julius is back in the hospital, they are doing a cat-scan now to check the extent of the staph infection. But Julius is expecting the worst and he's afraid to think about the sternum being infected. He doesn't think that he'll make it through the year (Journal, July 12, 2008).
>
> When the nice nurse on the 4th floor asked him how he described his health, he said poor—but then that he was just joking. But later, he said, "No, it was poor." That he'd never get out of the hospital. "I don't expect to recover—I just want to go home."
>
> Same day, 11:12 p.m.: Julius is much better, plus he's had some good care in the hospital on the 4th floor. The other thing is that the sternum doesn't seem to be an option for removal even if infected (Journal, July 19, 2008).

After receiving a pic-line in order to receive antibiotics, he was finally discharged from the hospital on July 21, 2008. His discharge report indicated that Julius did have osteomyelitis (infection of a bone) and it was the sternum; they would try to control it with antibiotics. Three days later, this approach seemed to be working as all his aches and pains were gone.

Bad Years, Good Years

The year 2008 was particularly difficult for Julius, with many hospital visits and stays. The following year was not quite as bad, although the infection on his right leg was not healing as his doctors had hoped:

> Julius's leg wound is almost healed, he was in pretty good spirits (Journal, March 20, 2009).
>
> Julius is back in the hospital, the pus underneath the leg wound scab looked awful. There was also a little hole and sudden bleeding. The ultrasound showed some murkiness from a deep sac of dead skin cells and blood that needed to be cut out (Journal, March 22, 2009).
>
> Julius is going in for surgery tomorrow morning, related to the little hole on his leg. The vascular surgeons got involved, too. Julius was in a good mood despite all this (Journal, March 25, 2009).
>
> Julius is ok and although the upper part of his leg looks good but it's swollen and huge. The cut from the amputation is to be left open as it is… (Journal, March 31, 2009).

After almost five months, his leg was sufficiently healed for Julius to get prepared to walk with two protheses:

> Julius was really happy, the plastic surgeon said that his leg wound is healing well, that he'll be fitted for a prosthesis soon, which will help him with his weight and also help him feel more independent (Journal, August 14, 2009).

The next five and a half years (2010 to mid-2015) were relatively good years for Julius, with very few hospital visits, in fact none in 2010 and 2011. He still had problems with low blood sugar incidents and one day, he passed out while riding one of Ann Arbor's AATA buses. But other than that incident, he was doing very well and was very happy living in his new house on Santa Fe Trail in Ann Arbor.

He was also pleased about his various University of Michigan presentations, events, and some of his classes:

> In January 2010, there was a book party celebrating the publication of the book, *The Origins of the Black Atlantic* (2010), co-edited by Laurent Dubois and Julius, which many people from the Department of History and DAAS attended (Journal, January 22, 2010).
>
> Julius's hand and arm were really hurting him last night. But he had fun shopping last night and his Coltrane class is FULL! (Journal, August 11, 2013).

Nonetheless, the continuing buildup of plaque in his arms led to more problems with his hands and in December 2014, he was in the hospital for tests and surgery. When the pain increased, his doctors insisted on surgery on January 1, 2015. While his hands continued to be painful, he was able to participate in a Department of Afroamerican and African Studies (DAAS) conference the following month:

> The Coltrane-Muhammed X session at the Department of Afroamerican and African Studies went well—and Julius was very happy. It was generally good and Julius's presentation was exceptional (Journal, February 20, 2015; Figure 4.2).

His participation in academic activities and invitations to present his work based on his dissertation research served as a sort of remedy which helped him to persevere with his diabetes.

Sense of Physical Decline

However, he had many medical challenges in the following years that undermined this confidence and contributed to his sense of decline and impending

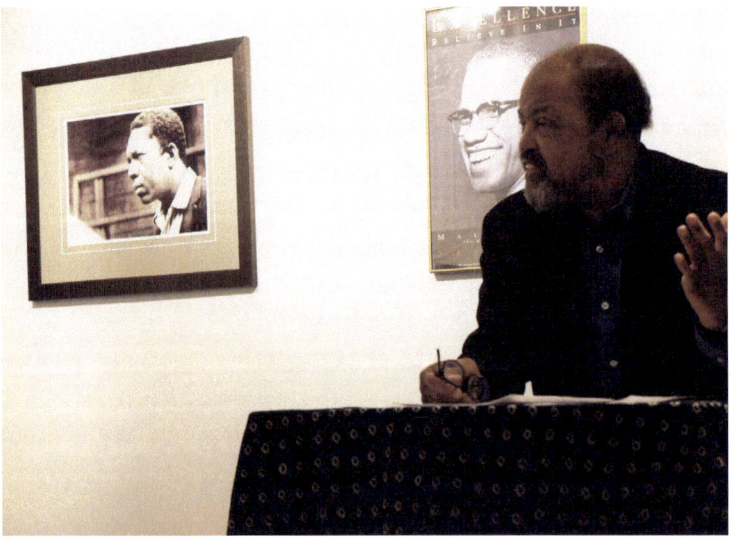

Figure 4.2. Julius presenting a talk on John Coltrane and Muhammed X at the Department of Afroamerican and African Studies, University of Michigan, Ann Arbor, Michigan, February 20, 2015; photograph by E.P. Renne.

death. Yet he had expressed his dismay with his experience of diabetes and the progressive deterioration of his body many years before.

> Julius said that when he was in the hospital, he would long for the four hours when they left him alone at night. Then he would cry for three hours, then compose himself in the final hour—to be his equanimous self. "Mr. Scott, you're so cheerful," whereas he'd been crying, "Why me?" (Journal, February 16, 2000).
>
> Julius still doesn't know what's what with his foot, he was very depressed last night. He just wants to quit (Journal, October 12, 2004).
>
> Julius said to his dog, Mogie, last night, "Which of us is going to die first? I'll die an early death" (Journal, February 2, 2006).
>
> Julius said tonight that he really doesn't care if his foot heals—"It's too late now." "Too late for what?" "I just don't care what happens, now, unlike last year" (Journal, September 27, 2006). [His foot was amputated on January 1, 2008.]
>
> Julius thinks that he surely is going to have another heart attack, which is what kills many diabetics. He actually had looked at actuarial accounts of those who'd had one (Journal, January 2, 2009).
>
> Julius said the saddest thing last night: "I'm not of any use to anyone" (Journal, September 2, 2009).
>
> Julius sat in his bed for a long time tonight. At one point he asked, "What if I died here—how long would it take you to notice?" "A couple of hours, I don't always come in your bedroom when you're asleep. And anyway, you're not going to die in your bedroom." "Where then—the hospital?" "No!" "Class?" "Maybe…" (Journal, October 28, 2009).
>
> At a restaurant last night, Julius was very out of it, not recognizing the server and talking to himself, "I'm not going to make it out of here" (Journal, December 29, 2009).
>
> Last night he said, "I might as well eat what I want, I don't have long to live, I could die tomorrow" (Journal, August 30, 2010).
>
> Julius had a nightmare and cried out in fear. It was about a stray cat in some sort of institution, a nunnery or mission, as there was a nun, whose head was bent down and when she lifted her head, her eyes were just whites—blank. She was death, looking at Julius. It was a terrifying nightmare (Journal, December 25, 2011).
>
> Julius is listening/watching a John Coltrane tape. He's engrossed and happy. This morning when asked if he thought he'd make it to 60 years old, he said, "No,

> but that if I do, I'll feel old and decrepit". But he doesn't feel that way at all now, he feels the same that he felt when he was young. So, despite all his health problems, he feels good (Journal, October 24, 2012).[2]
>
> Julius is doing fairly well, making urine. But he thinks that once he goes back on dialysis, it will be downhill (Journal, January 23, 2016).

Julius started hemodialysis at the DaVita clinic in Ann Arbor in the fall of 2015, which eventually became routine. He would get up at 5 a.m., quickly eat breakfast, and get dressed, in order to get to the clinic on time. Yet hemodialysis initially had some dangerous consequences for him:

> Julius had a terrible low blood sugar attack today, he was screaming and pushed himself out of his wheelchair. The paramedic said that these low blood sugar attacks have gotten worse because dialysis has thrown his system out of kelter. But Julius denied it. As he's been saying all along, it's just diabetes (Journal, April 16, 2016).

Depending on the state of his blood sugar equipment and medications he was taking, his blood sugar became increasingly difficult to control. The vagaries of his blood sugar led to the continuing buildup of plaque in his arms and hands:

> On one trip to Domino Farms, the doctor who looked at his hand wasn't very helpful or encouraging. Along with the leg sore, it seems to Julius as if his body is falling apart
>
> (Journal, June 16, 2017).

> This morning when changing his chest dressing, done once a day now that there is no discharge, he said, "Why bother? I'm going to die anyway" (Journal, February 9, 2018).
>
> Julius is in the ICU at Hilton Head Hospital, they've finally gotten his blood sugar down (it was 230) but he is still very disoriented if a bit better. While he could manage to have a conversation, he also said, "I think this will be the end" (Journal, March 30, 2019).

---

[2] In October 2012, he was 57 years old and, six years later, his book, *The Common Wind*, was published.

> Julius said something about a hallucination, that he deeply believed that they couldn't find a medicine that would prevent him from dying. But then he added that he wants his book to receive a prize (Journal, April 2, 2019).

His book, *The Common Wind: Afro-American Currents in the Age of the Haitian Revolution*, published in 2018, did indeed receive a prize, in fact, several prizes, as will be discussed in Chapter 5.

Yet his increasing disorientation, associated with diabetes, also contributed to his sense of physical decline:

> Yesterday Julius couldn't figure out how to add an email address to an email and couldn't figure out how to use the TV monitor. But today he reinstalled the blood sugar monitor and it worked so that was a huge improvement. In the discussion of the connection between diabetes and dementia, vascular cognitive impairment was also mentioned. So Dr. D's assessment was probably correct, that Julius just goes in and out of clear thinking, due to damage to the brain (Journal, April 27, 2019).
>
> Julius got up about 3:30 a.m. and sat in the kitchen, waiting for his breakfast. And before going for dialysis, he was in the laundry room but couldn't figure out how to put on his coat and was just standing there…So he's completely confused again (Journal, May 1, 2019).

Despite these setbacks, more surgeries on his hands, and challenges from his diabetes control equipment, he carried on:

> Julius is still good, he was in a much better mood yesterday too and even this morning was saying how thankful he was for not having Covid-19 (Journal, April 29, 2020).
>
> Julius is asleep, he's not looking well today. But they say he is doing well at dialysis and he's very pleased that he's lost weight (Journal, September 13, 2020).

And he was very happy to have his house on Santa Fe Trail:

> Julius was in a good mood yesterday. He was wheeling along the hallway and exclaimed, "I just love being in this house!" (Journal, June 24, 2020; Figure 4.3).

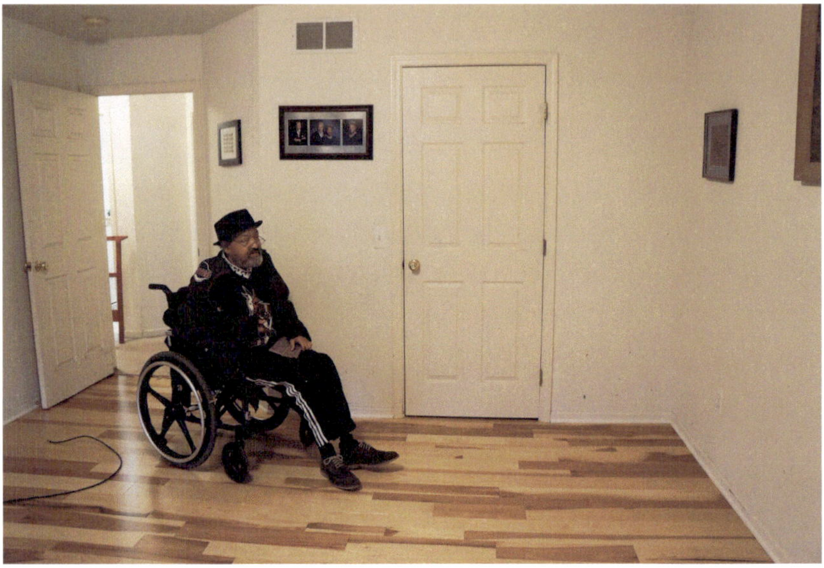

Figure 4.3. Julius was very pleased with the new wood floor that had been installed in his house, Ann Arbor, Michigan, April 9, 2016; photograph by E.P. Renne.

Final Stages of Diabetes

Julius was only in the hospital twice in 2020 although frequent episodes of low and high blood sugar continued. Some were due to problems with the G6 CGM meter that misfunctioned because blood had contaminated the glucose monitor sensor site, and sometimes the sensor would become disconnected. Then the sensor had to be replaced and finger-stick blood glucose readings taken. And as Julius had lost fingers on both hands, it became more and more difficult for him to insert a strip into the glucose monitor and then hold it when it registered his blood sugar. Despite these challenges, it was as if the good news about the publication of his book was positive medicine for him.

This happiness was followed by the appalling events in the final year of his life:

> Julius said that someone died while he was at dialysis. I think it was the older African woman, it must have been very disturbing for the new woman taking care of Julius. It was disturbing for Julius (Journal, March 22, 2021).
>
> Julius sounded so depressed, it is back to "it's too difficult, I may not make it" talk. But dialysis was ok today although his blood sugar was very

> high again. …This whole situation is impossible. He's thinking about death (Journal, May 27, 2021).

The ups and downs of his blood sugar, high temperatures caused by infections, increasing disorientation, and loss of balance led to three long hospital stays in November and early December 2021.

> Julius is in the ER at the hospital! He had low blood pressure, so low that they sent him to the hospital from the dialysis clinic. It's the first time he's been to the hospital for over a year. It's not clear what is causing this low blood pressure, if it has to do with diet or what (Journal, October 20, 2021).
>
> Julius sounded much better. They are giving him tests today to see why his blood pressure keeps going down at dialysis. He said it hasn't been bad when they take readings at home (Journal, October 28, 2021).

These low blood pressure readings continued, suggesting problems with his heart.

> Julius still hasn't received test results from his cardiologist. If the low blood pressure readings reflected a faulty machine at the dialysis clinic, he could consider going to the UM South Industrial dialysis site. "No," he replied, "It's not the machinery, it's my body." Yesterday wasn't too bad at dialysis but they are not taking off much fluid (Journal, October 30, 2021).

Indeed, it was a problem with his heart, which was related to his earlier coronary artery bypass surgery in 2008, his minor stroke also in 2008, and his cardiac arrest episode in 2015. Having long-term diabetes also contributed to problems with his heart.

> Julius is ok, but apparently he has a serious problem simply described as "a weak heart." His cardiologist said that his heart wasn't strong and is going to give him some medication and also look into the possibility of a pace-maker. But this would be six weeks after taking the medication. It is more serious than Julius wants to admit, but perhaps the pace-maker will help him. His mother told him that his father died from a weak heart. Julius said that his cardiologist had

> spoken at length with the physician's assistant at the DaVita clinic so they will be watching him during dialysis (Journal, November 5, 2021).

A week later, Julius was in the University of Michigan Hospital again, with problems related to his heart:

> Julius is in the ER-ICU, he's very out of it. This was after a long coughing spell so he went to the emergency room when it wouldn't stop. He barely recognized anyone once in the hospital (Journal, November 12, 2021).
>
> Julius is much better or at least he was yesterday. But he'll probably be ok after another night of rest and monitoring his temperature and blood pressure. It's unclear whether they've been able to identify the cause of his temperature and low blood pressure (Journal, November 13, 2021).

This situation led to the scheduling of more tests. While a hospital consultant advised a spinal MRI (magnetic resonance imaging), this test was dismissed by two University of Michigan doctors. But they did schedule a cardiac scan:

> Julius is still not back from his cardiac scan. He agreed to do it although it's taking longer than he was told. But then he's probably waiting for transport. He also was scheduled for catheter insertion for continued dialysis (Journal, November 17, 2021).
>
> Julius is finished with dialysis and had a pass on the cardiac scan. Also, a health care advisor from the hospital is going to talk with Julius tomorrow. Perhaps this hospital representative will see how all the trials and tribulations experienced by Julius undermined the healing process (Journal, November 18, 2021).
>
> Julius's blood sugar is over 300. They still are not giving him enough insulin (Journal, November 19, 2021).
>
> Julius is back in the hospital after his much-swollen hand caused the physician's assistant at the DaVita clinic much alarm (Journal, November 23, 2021).

Julius was discharged from the hospital so that he could come home for Thanksgiving. But he was breathing so heavily and was so sleepy, he couldn't eat his turkey dinner.

The next morning, he could not stand up. After going to the clinic for dialysis, he was told to return to the hospital, which he did.

> The hospital was ok, Julius was a bit better toward the end of the afternoon. But they still don't know why he has an infection and where it's located (Journal, November 27, 2021).
>
> Julius was much better this morning but got progressively worse as he got tired. After they moved him to an 8th floor room, he got much worse. It was as if they hurried him out of the Intensive Care Unit to the attic, getting rid of old patients who were not going to get better. But he did seem so much better this morning. Julius is worried and afraid. He knows that his situation is very tenuous (Journal, November 28, 2021).
>
> He's even worse today and didn't sleep last night. Furthermore, they misspoke about his having a night sitter and he pulled off the bandage on his leg. Really, it's unclear if he's going to make it. He's mumbling and keeps trying to pull off his catheter site connection. This is so horrible and there is very little support on the 8th floor, the place where they bring people to die (Journal, November 29, 2021).
>
> Julius is still awake and incoherent, although he can sort of respond to questions. The nurse came and gave him another Zolpidem [an oral sleeping tablet that dissolves under the tongue] and he said he slept a bit. But he's not really slept and just mumbled all night although he's not as jumpy as before (Journal, November 30, 2021).

The next six days included various efforts to improve Julius's condition, to no avail.

> All their tests and interventions aren't working, Julius is still so sick and not sleeping and not getting better. His family agreed that it was better for him to live without these ceaseless and painful interventions. So, he was moved to the 7th floor where doctors are providing Comfort Care—no more EGB [esophagogastroduodenoscopy], Lactulose [for constipation], taking blood/checking labs, and transfusions, only a few antibiotics to make him comfortable (Journal, December 5, 2021).

Julius died the following day, on December 6, 2021, at 12:48 a.m.

Conclusion

Diabetes is a terrible disease. Although there have been many improvements in monitoring blood sugar levels and dispensing insulin to maintain them within respectable limits, it is difficult for those with type 1 diabetes to live a long life with this condition. While Julius lost his lower legs, finger, and suffered from increasing heart problems, his academic research, publications, presentations, and awards countered the effects of his illness and provided him with great happiness in his final years.

On the advice of Marcus Rediker (University of Pittsburgh), the editor of Verso Press, Ben Mabie, contacted Julius about the possibility of publishing his PhD dissertation. While initially hesitant, his perfectionism raising doubts about revisions that he thought needed to be made, colleagues and friends convinced him to let Verso publish the dissertation "as is." Of course, he carefully read over the manuscript, even with his failing eyesight, and was kept busy with a small number of clarification questions from Verso. Polishing the manuscript for his book—and preparing for talks and presentations—was a therapeutic counter to the dangerous disease of diabetes. His book, *The Common Wind: Afro-American Currents in the Age of the Haitian Revolution*, is discussed in the following chapter.

Chapter 5
The Common Wind

> Though fallen thyself, never to rise again,
> Live, and take comfort. Thou has left behind
> Powers that will work for thee; air, earth, and skies;
> There's not a breathing of the common wind
> That will forget thee; thou hast great allies;
> They friends are exultations, agonies,
> And love, and man's unconquerable mind.
>
> William Wordsworth, "To Toussaint L'Ouverture," 1802

Julius Scott's study of the currents of communication among freed and enslaved Blacks in the Caribbean and the larger Atlantic world has been widely acclaimed as "an entirely new vision of a historical period...the age of revolution, one of the most profound moments in world history" (Rediker 2018: xxiii). The book's title makes reference to the sonnet honoring Toussaint L'Ouverture (an excerpt cited above), who led the Black residents of the island of Saint-Domingue (now known as Haiti) to follow the example of their French colonizers who sought for Liberté, Egalité, Fraternité in their homeland of France. Indeed, this French national motto is also the national motto of contemporary Haiti.

It is not surprising that the research for his book, based on his PhD dissertation, required extensive reading of books, manuscripts, documents, and letters, in archives and libraries in Haiti, Jamaica, Spain, the UK (London), and the United States, as Julius had always been a reader. Indeed, after he learned to read as a 6-year-old, he remembered hiding in the closet at night with a flashlight, reading books. As a primary school student in Houston, Texas (see Chapter 2), he received all As in his classes and went on to excel in the two private high schools he attended—Westminster in Atlanta and Indian Springs in Indian Springs Village, Alabama. He later went on to Brown University where he graduated in 1977 with *magna cum laude*, honors in history.

Reading the footnotes of his book, *The Common Wind*, underscores the diversity of his sources. Newspaper articles published in the late 18th century in Haiti (*Affiches americaines*, *Gazette officielle d'etat de Hayti*, *Nouvelles diverses*); in Jamaica (*Kingston Daily Advertiser*, *Royal Gazette*, *Savanna-la-Mar Gazette*); in London (*Morning Chronicle*); in Paris (*Gazette Nationale ou le Moniteur Universal*); and in the United States (in Boston, Philadelphia, Richmond), as well as in Barbados, Dominica, and Grenada, were often cited. Information from printed primary sources such as *Les papiers de General A.-N. de la Salle (Saint-Domingue 1792–93)* (Quimper: Imprimerie Ch. Cotonnec 1897); the twelve volumes of *La Revolution française et l'abolition de l'esclavage; Textes et documents* (Paris: Éditions d'histoire sociale, 1968); and the fourteen volumes of the *Journals of the Assembly of Jamaica* (A. Aikman and J. Lunan, 1811–29), were also incorporated into the text.

This research was conducted when Julius was a graduate student at Duke University, where many of the family papers that he utilized were held: for example, Joseph Villars Dubreuil (papers: 1760–1850), a French lieutenant colonel of the French Army, who was stationed in Santo Domingo; James Iredell (1751–1799), of North Carolina, one of the first US Supreme justices; and William Wilberforce (papers: 1759–1833), a leader in the British slave trade abolition movement. But it was several years earlier when he got to know Keith, his next-door neighbor and classmate in Atlanta, that he started to think about what it meant to be Black (Connolly 2022):

> The interesting thing about Keith was Keith's mother and family were from the Bahamas. He had grown up in Miami, but his mother had relatives in Atlanta. So when I went over to Keith's house, they were speaking pidgin. Each of these bright people was speaking a language that was really different.

Watching the 1968 Olympics with Keith, Julius began thinking about how to study Black people as not simply those living in Africa and in the United States—as he explained to his former student, Nathan Connolly, in 2021:

> In a way, watching those 1968 Olympics and hanging with Keith brought me increasingly toward this question: How were we related to people who looked

> like us, who lived in other places that were closer to us than Africa? What could we say about that particular relationship to make Black people better understood?
>
> There was a way we could understand connections between different, apparently disconnected places that helped us to bring together and understand something about each of these places on their own terms. That was something that was important to me. It would help all of us understand the Black world much better than we were being trained to understand it, as simply the US and Africa (Connolly 2021. Interview: Julius Scott, March 2021, Ann Arbor).

Julius's decision to pursue the study of the Haitian Revolution in the context of the connections and movements of people and ships in the Atlantic—both trans-European and Caribbean travels of and communication among sailors and traders—is what made his research and writing revolutionary itself. In order to think about Black people living in the Atlantic world more broadly, he began his research by thinking about Haiti. "I began thinking about, again, the questions that had been presented to me during the 1968 Olympics, seeing a wider Black world than just Africa versus the US."[1]

As it turned out, Julius's study of the racist responses of European political leaders and their efforts through blockades, trade embargoes, and ultimately the arrest and imprisonment of the leader of the revolution, Toussaint Louverture, underscored the success of the Haitian Revolution and Haitians who continued efforts to maintain their freedom. For as he notes in his book's epilogue: "Throughout the nineteenth and into the twentieth century, Afro-North Americans have derived inspiration from the example of Haitian freedom and maintained both direct and indirect contact with Haiti" (Scott 2018: 210).

Sailors, Slaves, and Communication

As an undergraduate, Julius observed that American history was taught in terms of specific places in the United States and their connections mainly with England. This perspective was not surprising, considering the ways that Afro-American history was largely ignored. Yet Afro-Americans played

[1] From Interview: Julius Scott, March 2021, by Nathan Connolly (2022).

an important role in US history: as soldiers in the Revolutionary army, as traders, and as field hands and domestic servants (more commonly known as slaves). However, he was anxious to provide a broader perspective that included the roles of people of the African diaspora in the Atlantic world—and to link places in the United States such as Charleston, South Carolina, and Philadelphia, Pennsylvania, with places in the Caribbean such as Jamaica and Saint-Domingue (Haiti).

As an admirer of the work of Fernand Braudel (1972), he wanted to examine connections in the Atlantic world as he told Nathan Connolly:

> I was so convinced by the ways that Braudel, with his vast knowledge, was able to really connect up the different areas that connected to the Mediterranean as a region. I said, well, the Caribbean is kind of like another Mediterranean, but even more so because there were so many different areas of the world or the history of the world that were connected to different places in the Caribbean.... And we had to understand those other places, as well as understand the ways particular places are related to each other, like Cuba is related to Jamaica and to Saint-Domingue.

Several years earlier (in 1987), Julius was most pleased to hear about Braudel in relation to his work in the Caribbean:

> When Julius went to UI-Circle Campus to give his job talk, he was taken to dinner by some members of the History Department and during dinner talk, he was told that there were some faculty members who didn't fully support an offer being made to him. In fact, he was warned about one notoriously critical faculty member, Professor X, who was known for the impossibly difficult questions he asked candidates at job talks. So the next day, after Julius presented his paper, he took questions which were basically informational. Then a man in the audience raised his hand and Julius called on him. "My name is X..." Julius remembered the warning he'd been given, nervously saying "Pleased to make your acquaintance," bracing himself for the question. X began: "I lived in France and was a friend of Fernand Braudel..." Julius kicked himself for trying to relate his work to that of Braudel. "And," he continued, "I want you to know that he would be proud and pleased to be associated with your work."

> Julius was hired by the History Department and later he and Professor X became colleagues and friends (Journal, November 13, 2018).

In order to encompass the Caribbean region as Braudel did for the Mediterranean, Julius focused on the knowledge, expertise, and movements of Black sailors, free Blacks, and Black slaves which enabled them to communicate news about the situations in places in the Caribbean as well as in Europe and the United States, pertaining to slavery and slave revolts. While many Blacks were unable to read (in part because of White Caribbean and US plantation owners' refusal to teach them reading in order to prohibit written communication[2]), information was spread by word of mouth and by combinations of news and rumors (Scott 2018: 78). Furthermore, fluency in several languages among Black sailors facilitated the spread of news—about the French Revolution, about British parliamentary discussions of the abolition of slavery, and about slave revolts throughout the Spanish Caribbean. Julius's own fluency in French and Spanish facilitated his research.

The Coming Out of *The Common Wind*

As has been discussed in Chapter 4, the publication of the book *The Common Wind* by Verso Press was an unexpected event. In 2016, when Julius's colleague, Marcus Rediker, was asked by the Verso editor, Ben Mabie, to recommend a manuscript for the press to publish, "Rediker had a very specific suggestion: 'You should publish *The Common Wind*,' he said" (Bartlett 2018). The following year when Julius was approached by the press, being the perfectionist that he was, he thought that it needed to be revised and updated:

> When he heard that Verso was interested in publishing *The Common Wind*, Scott was initially apprehensive.... "When I reread it, I noticed what I hadn't finished, or what I've come to understand better through the years," he says. His first impulse was to go back and try to add to the manuscript, to improve what seemed not quite right. Mabie, his Verso editor, talked him out of that (Bartlett 2018).

---

[2] Anti-literacy laws in the United States (Givens 2021).

Indeed, several people encouraged Julius to proceed with the book's publication, as a way of honoring his parents (which he did in the book's dedication). And Mabie encouraged him as well: "The book as it is, and the ground that it covers, it feels pretty exhaustive…We encouraged Julius to trust in the work he had done and bring it to press" (Bartlett 2018).

Julius agreed with the dissertation's publication as the book, *The Common Wind*, and in late December 2017, texted Marcus Rediker to thank him for the recommendation. "It's interesting, he wanted to tell his mother about it, he is so pleased" (Journal, December 9, 2017). Unfortunately, Julius continued to suffer from low blood sugar incidents, both at home and while at dialysis. Furthermore, in early January 2018, he still had not had word from Verso or Marcus about publication, so he wasn't sure about what was going on. But when he did hear details about the book's projected publication date, he was very happy (Journal, January 28, 2018).

Nonetheless, this happiness was tempered by more hospital stays, which had to do with his infected sternum (as was discussed in Chapter 4):

> Julius is back in the hospital, this time because of the opening of his chest scar and its suppuration. We went to the Emergency Room where he was admitted. But Julius is in good spirits. He is so glad about his book, Marcus Rediker wrote a wonderful foreword. It was read to Julius since it was unclear whether he could read long printed passages anymore (Journal, January 31, 2018).

Despite the five hospital stays in 2018—in January, February, July, and twice in August:

> Julius is working on his book chapters, he's almost finished, there aren't many corrections that need to be made (Journal, July 2, 2018).

Along with these corrections, work at Verso continued through the summer and early fall and on October 5, 2018, he received word that the book was ready to be sent. He was exuberant, although he was annoyed two weeks later that Verso had not sent him a sample copy. But the book had been sent to reviewers and on October 24, 2018, people from *The Chronicle Review* came to his house for an interview and photographs:

> There was a long session with the reviewer and photographer for the *Chronicle* piece on Julius and his book today. He was very pleased to have them to the house and they were both very nice. Many pictures were taken including some showing his hands with his missing fingers (Journal, October 24, 2018).
>
> The review of Julius's book, entitled, "An Underground Sensation Arrives," appeared in yesterday's *Chronicle Review*. He is thrilled and it is very good, both the article and the photographs (Journal, November 3, 2018; see Bartlett 2018).

There were several other reviews of his book, including in the *LA Review of Books* (Bressler 2019), in *The Nation* (Sinha 2019), in *The New York Review of Books* (Bell 2019), in *The Times Literary Supplement* (Hazareesingh 2019), and in *The London Review of Books* (Bhatia 2020), which pleased him immensely. And, as was noted in the University of Michigan History Department Newsletter:

> In February 2018, *TIME* magazine published "9 Books to Read for Black History Month, According to Scholars." Listed along with Ralph Ellison's *Invisible Man,* Michelle Alexander's *The New Jim Crow*, and W.E.B. Du Bois's *Black Reconstruction in America* was an unpublished doctoral thesis written at Duke University in 1986 by Julius S. Scott, who later became a University of Michigan faculty member in History and Afroamerican and African Studies. Since then, Dr. Scott's work, *The Common Wind: Afro-American Currents in the Age of the Haitian Revolution* [was published] by Verso (Parker 2019).

Julius was also glad to attend several events that celebrated the publication of his award-winning book. In March 2018, he attended the presentation, "The Maritime History of the Haitian Revolution: A Discussion with Julius Scott of his Forthcoming Book, 'The Common Wind,'" at the University of Pittsburgh. Then, in September 2019, he received the MAAH Stone Book Award, at the Museum of African American History in Boston, and in February 2020, the "Symposium on the Influence of Julius S. Scott's Writing and Teaching" was held at Duke University. Further announcements made Julius very happy, including another book award, The Franz Fanon Book Award for 2020, and the panel, "After the Common Wind: Atlantic Studies and the Work of Julius S. Scott III," held at the American Historical Association meeting in January 2019 in Chicago.

As a consequence of the favorable reviews, awards, and presentations, *The Common Wind* was sold out after its first printing. Following its reprinting and also publication as a paperback, the book was published in Spanish as *El Viento Comun* in 2021. Unfortunately, Julius did not live to see the Brazilian-Portuguese publication of his book projected to be published in 2024.

The Common Wind and Black History Month

In March 1991, Julius was interviewed by Dr. Caroline Lattimore as part of the series, "In Times Like These," associated with Duke University. Caroline was the first Black dean of minority affairs and Black assistant provost and Julius was an assistant professor in the Department of History at the time. They discussed a number of topics including the establishment of Black History Month, first conceived of as Negro History Week by the Black historian Carter Woodson in 1926 (Givens 2021; Mineo 2022). What motivated the establishment of this week (and later month) was the importance of Black agency, and the demand for American recognition of African Americans' contributions to US history.

However, Julius noted that Dr. Woodson was not the first African American historian in the United States to write about Black contributions to the history of the Black Atlantic world, citing John Russwurm and his Bowdoin College commencement speech in 1826. Russwurm was the first Black graduate of the college, located in Brunswick, Maine, and his speech was entitled "The Conditions and Prospects of Hayti" (Russwurm 2010; see also James 2010). Russwurm focused on the leading role of the country's military leader, Toussaint Louverture, and the importance of the Haitian Revolution, a theme that Julius took up in his own PhD dissertation. Julius noted, however, that while the American Revolution was widely taught in US elementary and secondary schools,[3] the Haitian Revolution was only infrequently mentioned.

Julius's interest in the connections between Black people living in the United States and the wider Black Atlantic world led him to think about connections between three interrelated revolutions during the late 18th century in the United States, in France, and in Haiti. Yet while the establishment of the United States as a country independent from Great Britain was celebrated

[3] There is not only little knowledge of Haitian history; eighth graders' US history test scores declined significantly in 2023 (Mervosh 2023).

in 1776 and the French people founded the French Republic in 1792 based on the equality of its citizens, the events associated with the Haitian Revolution are not widely known. Thus in France, as the former French prime minister and the head of France's Foundation for the Remembrance of Slavery, Jean-Marc Ayrault, noted: "A report published by the foundation in 2020 said that only one in 10 French primary and secondary school students learn about Louverture and the Haitian Revolution" (Méheut and Porter 2023).

And in the United States, this lapse in knowledge about the Haitian Revolution occurred despite the subsequent mass migration of White French plantation owners as well as Mulatto and Black refugees from Haiti after Black Haitian rebels overwhelmed French militia at Cap Français in 1793. Many came to the US coastal cities such as Charleston and Baltimore. However, southern US plantation owners, in particular, began to fear the importation of slave insurrections and rumors began to spread about the role of immigrants in such plans. These rumors led to the laws being enacted, beginning in South Carolina in 1794, "that made it illegal for any West Indian black to enter the state." North Carolina and Maryland soon followed suit (Scott 2018: 188–191).

While one might have assumed that with the end of slavery in Haiti initiated in 1791, in Jamaica in 1838, in the United States in 1865, and in Cuba in 1886, as well as with Toussaint Louverture declared as Governor-General in 1801 and with the independence of Haiti in 1804, that the conditions of Haitians and of Black people in the Atlantic world might have improved.[4] As the second independent nation in the "New World" (after the United States) and the first independent nation in Latin America and Caribbean, Haiti was also the first modern nation-state in the Atlantic ruled by people of African descent. As such it was an inspiration both to Blacks opposing slavery and inequality, and to those aspiring for post-colonial independence in other nations in the Americas. Yet the political situation in the United States—as evidenced by the 1794 law to limit Haitian Blacks emigrating to the Carolinas—and in France, where Napoleon Bonaparte sought to retake control of Haiti in 1802, made it very difficult for Haiti to recover from its extended battles for independence, as did subsequent obligations imposed on the country.

[4] It wasn't for another 46 years that France, on April 27, 1848, abolished slavery for a second and final time (Méheut and Porter 2023).

In the Epilogue of *The Common Wind*, Julius discusses the complicated relationship of the US and British governments with Toussaint Louverture and his government. While commercial trade through licensed ships officially was approved by the US and UK governments, there was considerable skepticism that Black sailors on Haitian vessels would refrain from instigating slave revolts in southern states in the United States and in Jamaica:

> "We may expect therefore black crews, and supercargoes and missionaries thence into the southern states," wrote Thomas Jefferson after President Adams lifted the embargo on trade with Saint-Domingue in 1799... Echoing Jefferson, British admiral Hyde Parker, commander on the Jamaica naval station, registered "strong objections ... against coloured communications" (Scott 2018: 204–205).

With recognition of Haiti's move toward independence by the United States and Great Britain, Toussaint agreed with the arrangements for the shared monopoly of Anglo-US ships regarding Haitian trade. However, despite Toussaint's cooperation, this monopoly was used to squeeze the Haitian economy, with "restrictions [that] limited tonnage and size of crews, and finally, prohibited any local vessel from sailing outside a radius of five leagues, or fifteen miles, of the coast" (Scott 2018: 206).

These strategies so weakened the Haitian economy and Toussaint's position that when Napoleon sent over 2,000 French soldiers, led by General Charles Leclerc, to Haiti in 1802, Toussaint was captured and sent to the French prison, Fort-de-Joux, in eastern France, where he died on April 7, 1803. Nonetheless, Haitian fighters were able to defeat Leclerc and the French militia, who surrendered in 1803, and on January 1, 1804, the new leader of Saint-Domingue, renamed Haiti, Jean-Jacques Dessalines, declared the country's independence.

Yet, while the nation of Haiti was finally recognized by France in 1825, this recognition came at exorbitant cost:

> In 1825, French warships returned and forced the young country to pay compensation for the colonial losses, or face war. Haiti became the world's first and only country in which the descendants of enslaved people paid reparations to the descendants of their masters, for generations. That debt, and the loans the country took out to pay for it, crippled the country's economy for more than a century (Méheut and Porter 2023).

An extensive investigation conducted by *New York Times* reporters and researchers in 2021–2022 found numerous primary documents in Haiti and France from the late 1700s and 1800s that enabled them to estimate, with considerable accuracy, the debt (or ransom as Porter et al. 2022a describe it) placed on Haiti by France.[5] Their investigation:

> revealed that over six decades, Haiti sent $560 million in today's dollars to descendants of former colonists and the banks that offered the first loan. Had that money stayed in the country, it would have grown the economy from $21 billion to $115 billion over two centuries. And that does not include later loans taken out (Méheut and Porter 2023).

By threatening to invade Haiti again—as French officers had attempted in 1802—the Haitian Government conceded to the French demand. Yet "the amount was far beyond Haiti's meager means. Even the first installment was about six times the government's income that year, based on official receipts documented by the 19th-century Haitian historian Beaubrun Ardouin" (Porter et al. 2022a). Subsequently, the Haitian Government was forced to take out loans from French banks, which they were eventually forced to pay back with interest.

> This became known as Haiti's "double debt"—the ransom and the loan to pay it—a stunning load that boosted the fledgling Parisian international banking system and helped cement Haiti's path into poverty and underdevelopment.... The double debt helped set off a cascade of privation, budgetary shortfalls and onerous foreign loans that shaped the country into the 20th century and beyond (Porter et al. 2022a; Nagourney 2022).

This "double debt" continued until 1888, when Haiti officially made its final payments. Nonetheless, the government still needed funds and in 1874 and 1875 took out two additional loans (Gamio et al. 2022).

However, this economic exploitation of Haiti was continued by the US Government. America had long been opposed to the independence of Haiti and only recognized it as a nation-state in 1862, when the southern states

---

[5] See Porter et al. (2022b) for a detailed discussion of the methods and materials associated with this study. *The Common Wind: Afro-American Currents in the Age of the Haitian Revolution* by Julius Scott is cited in this article.

seceded from the United States, just prior to the civil war. US politicians put pressure on the government to push France out and to invade Haiti in order "to prevent European intervention in the Western Hemisphere..., an action justified under the Monroe Doctrine" (*Encyclopedia Britannica* 2023). Yet Wall Street was extremely interested in US control of Haiti as reflected by the takeover of funds from the National Bank of the Republic of Haiti in December 1914:

> Eight American Marines strolled into the headquarters of Haiti's national bank and walked out with $500,000 in gold, packed in wooden boxes. They drove the loot by wagon to the shore, past American soldiers in civilian clothes who kept watch along the route. Once at the water, they loaded the boxes and sped to an awaiting gunboat. The gold was in the vault of a Wall Street bank within days (Gebrekidan et al. 2022).

In the summer of 1915, American troops began the US military occupation of Haiti which lasted until 1934. This invasion was deemed obligatory since:

> The country was so poor and unstable, the explanation went, that if the United States didn't take over, some other power would—in America's backyard, no less. Secretary of State Robert Lansing also portrayed the occupation as a civilizing mission to end the "anarchy, savagery and oppression" in Haiti, convinced that, as he once wrote, "the African race are devoid of any capacity for political organization" (Gebrekidan et al. 2022).

Yet the United States continued financial control of the country, directly and then indirectly, until 1947.

Afro-American Currents in the Atlantic World: Crossing Boundaries in Place and Time

The economic struggles that faced the Haitian people as a consequence of French and American exploitation have left the country impoverished and politically unstable. The current situation in Haiti—with political uncertainty and violence—reflects its earlier history. For on July 7, 2021, the president of Haiti, Jovenel Moïse, was murdered in his home outside of Port-au-Prince and "prosecutors say the plot to overthrow and ultimately kill him was hatched in South Florida by businessmen who hoped to reap lucrative contracts under a new administration" (Abi-Habib et al. 2023). Subsequent investigation by the US Government has led to the arrest of eleven people in the United States and "more than a dozen in Haiti for suspected ties to the assassination."

> Among those detained and indicted by a federal grand jury in South Florida on Tuesday were Antonio Intriago, a Venezuelan American, and Arcángel Pretel Ortiz, a Colombian living in the United States, the owners of a U.S. security company who prosecutors say organized the plot to murder the former Haitian leader.
>
> The assassination of the 43rd President Jovenel Moïse in July 2021, continues to leave Haiti in a dangerous political condition, with no president officially installed (Abi-Habib et al. 2023).

Along with this assassination, which has left Haiti with an unpopular acting prime minister, Ariel Henry, violent gangs marauded the streets of Port-au-Prince, making the basic requirements of life—food, water, and health care—dangerous to come by (Polgreen 2022). Their presence, associated with the presidency of Jean-Bertrand Aristide, who went into exile in 2004, reflects the complicated political story of contemporary Haiti. For example, "Aristide had made powerful enemies. He had demanded that France pay Haiti $21 billion, recompense for the repugnant debt it placed on its now liberated colony. The French were among the first nations to demand his ouster" (Polgreen 2022). However, as the *New York Times* journalist, Lydia Polgreen (2022), has observed:

> The best of what he [Aristede] represented—a demand for just redistribution, from without and within, as a route to true democracy and equity, was gone. What remained was his worst impulse: the gangs that had helped secure his presidency. It was a trauma from which Haiti has never really recovered, leaving it a broken nation living in the shadow of the most powerful country in the world.

Following the murder of President Moïse, some have suggested that the United States should intervene to restore peace to Haiti, although US President Biden has declined to do so (Crowley et al. 2021). However, Haitian immigration to the United States has been facilitated to some extent by a plan that "expands the use of a government app for migrants to apply for … a legal pathway for people from Cuba, Haiti, Nicaragua and Venezuela to be eligible for a two-year parole in the United States" (Sullivan and Fisher 2023). However, emigration is not the solution for restoring the vitality of the Haitian nation.

Remembering the Past and Toussaint Louverture

Despite the current difficulties and dangers in Haiti, there is some hope that together, many Haitians may bring about the emergence of a politically viable and peaceful nation:

> A broad swath of Haitian society, including rival political parties, trade unions, grass-roots community groups and human rights activists, have come together to propose a detailed framework for a political transition. Their compact, called the Montana Accord, calls for an appointed interim president, and the members of the group elected a former Haitian central bank governor named Fritz Jean as a consensus candidate for the job early this year (Polgreen 2022).

Perhaps the memories of Toussaint Louverture will remind people to respect Haiti's past and to allow Haitians to remake their present and prepare for their future. For as Polgreen (2022) notes: "The first step to helping Haiti fulfill its destiny, to be the independent Black republic its revolution promised, may be for the rest of us to get out of its way." Nonetheless, some form of reparations for the damage done by slavery and subsequent French "debt" and loans would certainly facilitate this process.

Macron Honors Toussaint Louverture

On April 27, 2023, the President of France, Emmanuel Macron paid tribute to Toussaint Louverture in the French prison where he died in 1803. "Toussaint Louverture strove to give life to the Declaration of the Rights of Man and of the Citizen," Mr. Macron said in a speech delivered on the 175th anniversary of France's abolition of slavery. "That which offered freedom, equality, fraternity to all" (Méheut and Porter 2023).

Macron's presence was the first time that a French political leader came to the prison to make an official statement in order to reconcile France with its colonial past. However, Macron did not mention the payments that France forced Haiti to make in compensation to former slave owners beginning in 1825. "The simple fact of pronouncing this name, Toussaint Louverture, is therefore a reparation for the affront made to a great Frenchman," Macron said.

Others have taken a different position on this perspective. Thus, while Macron's recognition of France's role in slavery and colonial rule in Haiti is admirable, as Karfa Diallo, the founder of Memories and Sharing,[6] has said, "France cannot 'pay tribute to Toussaint Louverture while ignoring Haiti's demands for justice' " (Méheut and Porter 2023).

It is important to note that "several prominent scholars, activists and politicians in both France and Haiti have long called on France to return the money," including Jean-Marc Ayrault, the former French prime minister. And Leslie Voltaire, a former Haitian official, welcomed the tribute but said France owed Haiti more than words. "Mr. Voltaire pointed out that a former French president, François Hollande, had promised to repay that debt in 2015. 'I would have liked to hear a follow-up to that,' he said" (Méheut and Porter 2023).

Conclusion

In *The Common Wind*, Julius Scott documents the many people working and traveling on ships throughout the Caribbean who contributed to the Haitian Revolution. In many small ways—word of mouth, rumors, and group readings of antislavery pamphlets—they transferred knowledge about political events on the island and throughout the Atlantic world. For as Malkah Bressler (2019) has written regarding Julius's perspective on colonial rule in the Caribbean:

> Scott argues…that commerce and trade also brought about the downfall of the colonial system in the Caribbean. First of all, trade required mobile people to transport goods and load and unload ships…. As these people traveled throughout the Caribbean trading material goods and human beings, their

[6] A French organization that campaigns for greater recognition of France's slavery and colonial past.

> commercial enterprises allowed for conversations. Thus, news and information were exchanged as well. The information traveled via transatlantic ships, inter-island sailing vessels, and through legal and illegal trade. As a result, news spread rapidly, despite colonial efforts to limit the spread of information. In fact, thanks to trade, enslaved peoples and free people of color were sometimes better informed than colonial officials and plantation owners.

In his interview with Dr. Caroline Lattimore in 1991, Julius made a similar point about beneficial changes in the lives of African Americans in the United States. Rather than focusing solely on the important exemplary and famous Black political leaders such as Martin Luther King Jr. and John Lewis, people need to recognize the small everyday ways that Black people improved their standing in the country. "For example, the Black student who was among the first to integrate an all-White school in the South, who got all A's and was best in their class, that was also a way of change," Julius noted.

Yet while the less well-known actions of sailors and traders in supporting the Haitian Revolution were vitally important, the first president of Haiti, Toussaint Louverture, remains a leading figure known for promoting Black leadership in the Atlantic world:

> Nineteenth-century Afro-North American historians like ex-slave William Wells Brown characterized the revolution in Saint-Domingue as a pivotal event in the history of Afro-Americans. . . . Up to the present day, Toussaint and the Haitian Revolution continue to occupy a central place in the cultural memory of blacks in North America (Scott 2018: 211).

In his book, *The Common Wind*, Julius underscores the importance of remembering the history of Black people and their efforts to stand up for justice and equality in Haiti, in the United States, and elsewhere in the Caribbean. Indeed, the issues raised by the Haitian Revolution discussed in the book are related to past actions such as Haitian leaders' offer of asylum to Simon Bolivar in 1817 and Toussaint Louverture as an inspiration for Denmark Vesey's rebellion in South Carolina (Scott 2018: 209–210), as well as to current US issues (e.g., racism, fear of immigrants, economic inequality, and attempts to address political power ploys). Indeed, while being honored in France, Toussaint Louverture continues to be a revered ancestor of Black people in the Caribbean and in the wider Atlantic world,

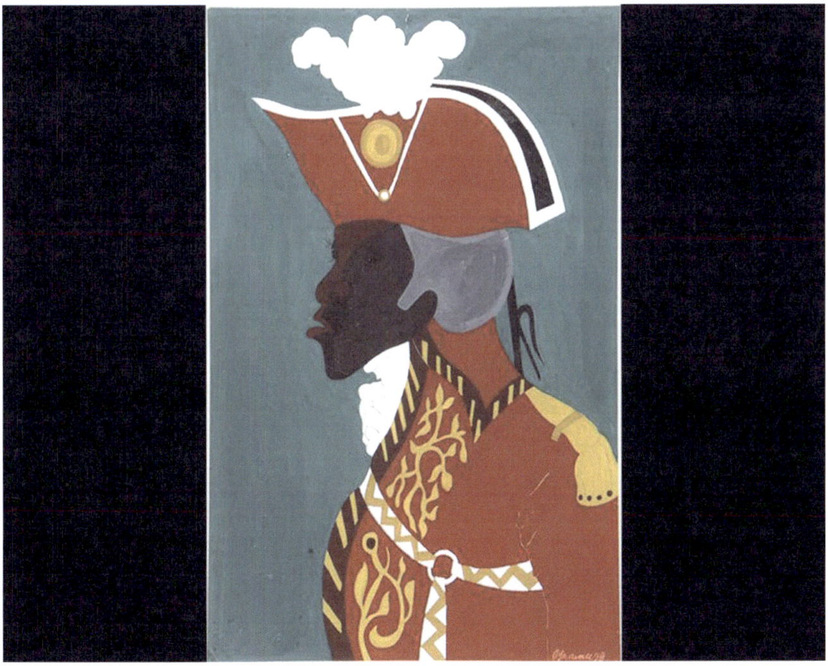

Figure 5.1. Toussaint L'Ouverture, print by Jacob Lawrence, 1938 (Courtesy of the Amistad Research Center, New Orleans, LA/ Bridgeman Images).

evidenced by the Latin rock band, Santana's, performance of their song, "Toussaint L'Ouverture" (released in 1971); by the fifteen prints by Jacob Lawrence (made in 1986–1997) depicting *The Life of Toussaint L'Ouverture* (Figure 5.1); and by the poem, "Toussaint," by Ntozake Shange (published in 1997; Scott 2018: 211).

While his great admiration for Toussaint Louverture is evident in his book, Julius Scott focuses on the informal news and information transmission—"the regional network of communication—the 'common wind'"—of common people. How such communication may be reinterpreted in the 21st century—perhaps through improved global internet access—within contemporary Caribbean societies in ways that may improve equality and justice remains to be seen.

In *The Common Wind*, there is a brief mention of the late 18th-century Caribbean trader, Isaac Sasportas (Scott 2018: 204). Isaac Sasportas conducted business throughout the Atlantic Caribbean area and was executed in Kingston, Jamaica, in 1799 as a spy plotting to incite a slave rebellion. While Julius submitted his research on Sasportas to the journal, *Annales,* this work remains unpublished. However, writing this manuscript—and thinking about the issues raised by the life of Sasportas and his world—was a therapeutic counter to the continuing health problems related to diabetes. Julius's manuscript, "Haitian Revolution and Sasportas's Jamaican Conspiracy, 1799," may be read in the following chapter.

Chapter 6

The Haitian Revolution and Isaac Sasportas's Jamaican Conspiracy

While his dissertation, *The Common Wind: Currents of Afro-American Communication in the Era of the Haitian Revolution*, was officially submitted to the Department of History at Duke University on July 18, 1986, Julius did not stop thinking about issues related to the mobility of people in the Caribbean during the late 18th and early 19th centuries. Indeed, he continued to examine his extensive archival data for further details about how their movements and the information that they shared contributed to other instances of Black insurrection in the Caribbean world. One such attempt, initiated by Isaac Sasportas—a young man associated with France but of several national affiliations in the Caribbean—is mentioned by Julius in a paragraph in his book's epilogue:

> Later that year [1799], the longstanding fears of white Jamaicans that the rebels in Saint-Domingue would export their revolution "by the help of the magick word Liberty" were almost realized. In December 1799, British officials executed Isaac Sasportas, a Jewish merchant from Saint-Domingue and partisan of the revolutions in France and the Caribbean, after finding him guilty of infiltrating the island in order to rally black support for an invasion from Saint-Domingue (Scott 2018: 204).

In the paper that he subsequently wrote in 2000, Julius considered the movements and people whom Sasportas interacted with, rather than specifically focusing on the details of his life. He presented his paper in several places: at a lecture at Hartwick College, Oneonta, New York, in November 2000; at the Latin American Studies Association meeting, Dallas, in 2003 ("Revolutionary Diaspora: Jews and the Revolution in Saint-Domingue");

and at a conference on "The Haitian Revolution in Global Perspective," held at Cornell University, Ithaca, New York, in 2004 ("Saint-Domingue and the Revolutionary Imagination of the 1790s: The Case of Isaac Sasportas"). An edited, unpublished version of the manuscript from 2002 follows.

The Haitian Revolution and Sasportas's Jamaican Conspiracy, 1799

Julius S. Scott

Beginning late in December, 1799, newspapers from Kingston to New York reported the public execution of a man "who had been found on the island of Jamaica under such circumstances as subjected him to conviction as a spy."[1] The suspect, found guilty of plotting an insurrection of disaffected elements on the British island, had been hanged a couple of days before Christmas in front of an approving crowd in the Kingston parade. "Conducted with the utmost solemnity," the ritualized execution began just after four o'clock in the afternoon. Secured in the custody of the Kingston militia, the prisoner was marched in irons from the guard house, then once around the square, with the labels "SPY" and "ESPION" attached respectively to his breast and back. The prisoner then climbed the ladder up to the scaffold platform, where a handkerchief was tied about his head, the noose fitted around his neck, and his body hanged until he died. The convicted conspirator's lifeless corpse was then drawn and quartered.

The newspaper stories agreed on these basic facts, but important particulars—and the "spin" locating the executed spy by identity, by politics, and in geographic space—remained contested and debated. Some claimed that "the spy lately hung at Kingston, Jamaica" was none other than "the Frenchman 'Sasportas,'" a notorious Jacobin "who in 1792, 1793, and 1794 was noted as the agent for French privateers at Charleston." Others implicated this "gentleman of considerable fortune and great worth" in "the memorable riot" in Charleston in 1793 "denominated the 'Riot at the Theatre,'" in which unsuspecting citizens out for a night attending a play were forcibly "driven

[1] See the stories of this execution and reprints of accounts from competing newspapers in Philadelphia in the *Gazetteer of the United States*, February 17, 1800, and in the Philadelphia *Aurora and General Advertiser*, February 22, 1800. The eyewitness account upon which these stories were partially based appeared in the *Kingston Royal Gazette*, December 28, 1799.

from the theatre" by a belligerent contingent of French sailors and sympathizers "with drawn daggers."

The predictably anti-French tenor of such Federalist accounts prompted the opposition Republican press to propose a quite different explanation of the Jamaica execution. The *Philadelphia Aurora* presented the convicted conspirator to be neither a Charlestonian nor a "Frenchman," but instead "a man of colour of the island of St. Domingo" whose name was not even Sasportas but "Das Portas." The latter account shifted the probable source of the conspiracy away from white partisans of the French Revolution, attributing the attempt on Jamaica not to stubborn Jacobins left over from the early 1790s but rather to the revolution of African slaves and free people of color in Jamaica's troubling neighbor, the French colony of Saint-Domingue. By 1800, Saint-Domingue had been in revolt for almost a decade, slavery had been outlawed in this and other French Caribbean territories for six years, and the rebellious colony on the island of Hispaniola was moving toward independence from France under black and brown leadership—with an as yet undetermined politics toward its anxious slaveholding neighbors, including the United States. Throughout the 1790s, slaveholders from Charleston to Caracas had detected symptoms of a Caribbean "contagion of liberty" spreading northward.

Both explanations proved more accurate reflections of competing political agendas in a heated election year than insight into the details of the 1799 Jamaica conspiracy. The executed man, one Isaac Jesurun Sasportas, manages to elude the categories of political description employed by the contending sides—whereby individuals involved in sedition in the late 1790s were likely to be connected either to France or to a French colony. Sasportas turned out to be neither the radical French immigrant of Federalist imagination nor the insurgent colored man depicted in Republican portrayals, and something more than a combination of those two images. Where these North American profiles diverged from documented details recoverable from other sources is worth noting. First, Sasportas's activities and connections ranged much more widely than the Philadelphia newspapers reported. A well-known gambler who frequented gaming tables in Cuba, Jamaica, and Saint-Domingue by night, a specialist in the active and often illicit traffic linking those islands by day, Sasportas had no fixed place of address. He was a longtime occasional resident of several imperial outposts—St. Thomas, Santiago de Cuba, and Cap Français—who was carrying Danish, Spanish, and French papers at the time of his arrest (Map 6.1).

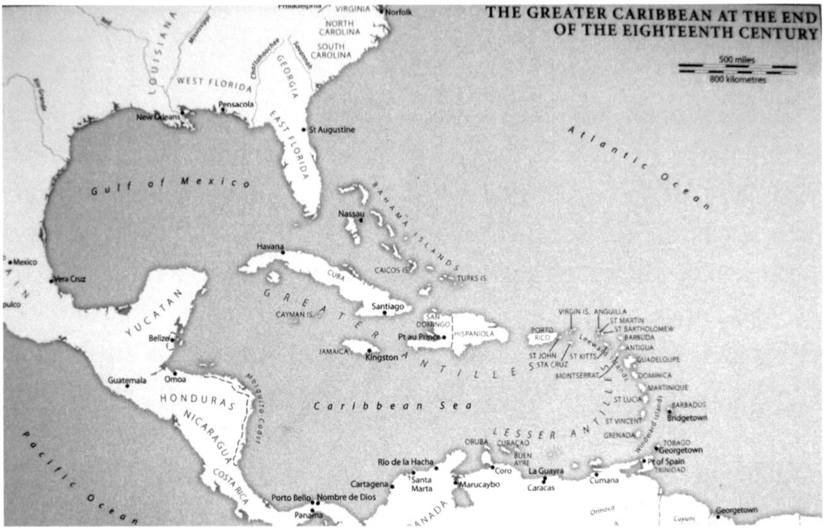

Map 6.1. Map of the greater Caribbean at the end of the 18th century (in *The Common Wind: Afro-American Currents in the Age of the Haitian Revolution*, by Julius Scott, 2018, p. xxi; New York: Verso Press). Reproduced with permission of the Licensor through PLSclear.

He claimed a similarly scattered network of kin that extended all over the Atlantic basin—from Dutch Curaçao to Europe. Sasportas never served as a French privateering agent in Charleston, but his uncle, Abraham Sasportas, whom Isaac visited on occasion, did. The joint Federalist-Republican portrait of Sasportas proved inaccurate in one other significant respect: despite his ties to Saint-Domingue, he was not a man of color but of Jewish heritage.[2] Even today—just as 200 years ago—this aspect of this radical's identity appears at least to be surprising. This essay, less concerned with recounting the details of the Jamaica plot, aims instead to reconstruct some of the contours of Sasportas's world. That reconstruction highlights both the utility

[2] Examination of Isaac Sasportas, November 19, 1799, with "Proceedings of a Court Martial held by virtue of a Special Commission," Spanish Town, December 16–17, 1799, Colonial Office 137/103, Public Record Office, Kew (hereafter C.O., PRO); G. Debien and P. Pluchon, "Un plan d'invasion de la Jamaique en 1799 et la politique anglo-americaine de Toussaint Louverture," *Revue de la Societe Haitienne d'Histoire, de Geographie et de Geologie* 36 (Juillet 1978): 112–13. For Abraham Sasportas, see James William Hagy, *This Happy Land: The Jews of Colonial and Antebellum Charleston* (Tuscaloosa and London: University of Alabama Press, 1993), 20, 92, 95, 118, 180; Charles Reznikoff, *The Jews of Charleston: A History of an American Jewish Community* (Philadelphia: Jewish Publication Society of America, 1950), 69; Barnett A. Elzas, *The Jews of South Carolina from the Earliest Times to the Present Day* (Philadelphia: J.B. Lippincott, 1905), 106, 242; Eugene Perry Link, *Democratic Republican Societies, 1790–1800* (Morningside Heights, NY: Columbia University Press, 1942), 87; and Melvin H. Jackson, *Privateers in Charleston, 1793–1796: An Account of a French Palatinate in South* Carolina (Washington, DC: Smithsonian Institution Press, 1969), 58, 69–71, 73n, 93.

of, and some of the problems presented by, approaching this rather obscure episode of late 18th-century radicalism within the framework of "Atlantic history." Sasportas's Jamaican conspiracy, in the end unsuccessful, attempts to mount fundamental challenges to social orders based on slavery that punctuate the era of the Haitian Revolution in the Americas. Exposed well before everything was in place, the projected uprising never took place. But, particularly at this time of polemical and often ahistorical discussion of the relationship between descendants of Africans and Jews—discussion that has at times focused on the role of Jews in American slavery—taking a close look at even such an abortive effort poses a host of interesting new questions.

Isaac Sasportas and French Plans to Destabilize Jamaica

The roots of the Jamaican conspiracy of 1799 seem to have several sources that suggest a range of influences—political, imperial, and personal. In the spring of 1799, Isaac Sasportas, a young man in his early to mid-twenties, approached French officials in Cap Français with a plan to destabilize Jamaica, Saint-Domingue's neighbor and the most valuable and strategically important British colony in all of America. "Since the dawn of liberty," his petition began, "I have been devoted to my Country." Animated to serve "with brilliance, with honor and passion," Sasportas petitioned Phillipe Roume, Special Agent of the Directory, to support his attempt to "plant... the tricolor flag" in the "very heart" of the British empire or die in the effort. He would travel to Jamaica and take political soundings there in an effort to "raise the army" of "converts" to the French cause. For three years, Sasportas intimated, "I have nourished in my heart the hope of avenging the friends the British sacrificed." Sasportas promised a detailed report demonstrating "ways of achieving the ends that I am proposing." The young merchant, conversant in English and knowledgeable of the "customs" of the British island from visits there, saw himself for these reasons as the optimal person to take on what he called "this great work." Within a couple of days of receiving Sasportas's letter, Roume arranged an evening meeting at his residence that included Sasportas as well as adjutant-general Devaux, a French military official.[3]

[3] Isaac Sasportas to Philippe Roume, 22 germinal, an 7, in "Depech de L'agent Roume au ministre du germinal, an 8—project de soulevement á la Jamaique," AOM, Colonies, CC 9B/17.

French plans to destabilize Jamaica somehow had been rumored among officials in the British West Indies as well as discussed openly and in secret by a variety of supporters of France since news of the French declaration of war against Great Britain had first arrived in the Americas in 1793. As early as April 1795, British officials foiled an alarming "attempt to set fire to Kingston," which they attributed to a far-reaching conspiracy. This conspiracy included fractious elements among the hundreds of French-speaking refugees from the insurrection in Saint-Domingue; "multitudes" of French prisoners of war "released from their confinement [and] let loose on Parole;" and various nameless "Emissaries"—including among their number "Mulattoes and Negroes from St. Domingo"—who, according to the newly appointed lieutenant governor of the island, had "succeeded in Landing their incendiaries" in an attempt to insurrect the colony.[4] Three months later, a fire destroyed what one official called "the most valuable part" of the north coast town of Montego Bay, including "a good deal of the powder and artillery of the militia" and tons of "Produce, Provisions, Lumber, and Supplies that were deposited at the different wharves." The Montego Bay fire was deemed accidental, but barely a month later, some 300 maroons and runaway slaves in neighboring Trelawny and Accompong took up arms and tried to appropriate "the dominion of this Country." Officials again charged that "Emissaries from the French had been in the Country of the Maroons" and that such men "of most dangerous description" lurked "at the bottom of this Business."[5] So there were both real and imagined antecedents, recent ones, to Sasportas's suggesting that Jamaica be targeted.

While Sasportas's original petition did not refer explicitly to any other aspect of his identity besides his French citizenship, Roume later recalled a striking new motive that emerged in their discussion: the eager young man's hope and desire that his actions would help to "wash away the stain that disgraces the Jewish nation of which he is a part." A successful mission, as its details became known to the world, would help to "prove to the human

---

[4] See Lord Balcarre's "Private and most Confidential" letter to an unidentified correspondent, May 3, 1795, MS 606, National Library of Jamaica, Institute of Jamaica, Kingston (hereinafter NLJ-IJ); and Balcarres to Duke of Portland, May 30, 1795, C.O. 137/95, PRO. By the spring of 1795, officials counted more than two hundred families of Saint-Domingue refugees in Jamaica, almost half of whom received government assistance. See Balcarres to Adam Williamson, April 27, 1795, and Balcarres to Portland, May 30, 1795, C.O. 137/95, PRO.

[5] Balcarres to Duke of Portland, June 10, July 19, July 23, August 25, 1795, C.O. 137/95, PRO.

race" that Jews were worthy of the "respect and the confidence of the French people."[6]

Over the next eight months, the circle of interest and involvement in Sasportas's project steadily widened to include a variety of French military officials, and partly due to Sasportas's own indiscretion, word that the French were planning to strike Jamaica began to surface in places outside Saint-Domingue, even as Roume and others in the colony moved forward in what they thought was careful secrecy. These officials found a partner for Sasportas, one Barthélemy Dubuisson, a lowly army officer and reluctant conspirator whom they forced to participate in order to make up for a brief traitorous collaboration with enemy forces during Britain's five-year annexation and occupation of much of eastern Saint-Domingue.

As for Sasportas himself, design and chance combined to deposit him in Jamaica sooner than expected. In May 1799, Sasportas boarded the French ship *Espérance*, a vessel in which he held a partial interest, in order to travel to St. Thomas to settle some business before turning his attention to the project. Just out of Cap Français, however, the vessel on which Sasportas was traveling was taken by the British cruiser, *Sprightly*, and brought into Port Royal, Jamaica, as a prize. Sasportas and the other passengers and crew were set at liberty in Kingston while a Vice-Admiralty court determined whether the prize was lawful. Left to his own devices, Sasportas inquired after the whereabouts of a particular Black man named Charles, who was to serve as his principal contact in Jamaica. Back in 1785, Charles had been purchased in Jamaica as a slave by Sasportas's father, a resident of Saint-Domingue, and taken to the French island to work for him. Five years later, Charles escaped, returned to Jamaica, and found employment serving aboard plantain boats engaged in local commerce. Sasportas had last spoken to Charles in Jamaica during his stay there in 1797, but now he hoped to depend on his father's former slave to get him in touch with maroons and other possible collaborators in the island's masterless underground.[7]

---

[6] Roume to Minister of the Marine, 2 germinal, an 8, ADM, Col., CC/17.

[7] For the circumstances of Sasportas's capture, see the examination of François Ferand, May 18, 1799, in papers of L'Espérance, JHCVA Papers, JA [Jamaica Archives, Spanish Town Jamaica—Records of the Jamaica High Court of Vice-Admiralty, 1793–1799]. See also the relevant sections of "Proceedings of a Court Martial held by virtue of a Special Commission," December 16, 1799, C.O. 137/103, PRO, and Isaac Sasportas to Toussaint Louverture, 30 Vendemiaire, an 8 (October 2, 1799), copy in C.O. 137/103, PRO.

Charles was well aware of the progress of the Saint-Domingue revolution, revealed by Sasportas months later in a report submitted to the rebel leader Toussaint Louverture to apprise him of the preparations for what French officials began to call the "descent" on Jamaica. Building on Charles's admiration for Toussaint, Sasportas promised "all the help imaginable" in the coming revolt. Charles in turn "promised me for his part to work to prepare spirits."[8]

In the months leading up to November 1799, an elaborate plan developed that involved two stages. First, an uprising of disaffected people in the island itself, spearheaded by maroons and joined by French refugees, thousands of whom had crowded into Kingston and the surrounding area between 1793 and 1798, when the British abandoned their effort to annex and occupy Port-au-Prince and the eastern coast of Saint-Domingue. The projected second stage involved the landing at Port Antonio of as many as 4,000 armed troops from Saint-Domingue to take advantage of the prevailing chaos and establish French control. Sasportas told the lieutenant governor after his arrest that the goal was to institute "universal liberty" on the island.

Sasportas arrived via Santiago de Cuba in November 1799. He met Dubuisson in Kingston, but the two of them were arrested only days after his arrival. Toussaint Louverture passed word to British officials of the presence and mission of Sasportas and Dubuisson for complex political reasons. [In the Epilogue of *The Common Wind*, Julius discusses this complicated relationship of the British and US governments with Toussaint Louverture and his government. With the recognition of Haiti's move toward independence, commercial trade through licensed ships officially was approved by Great Britain and the United States and Toussaint subsequently agreed with the arrangements for the shared monopoly of Anglo-US ships regarding Haitian trade (Scott 2018: 204–206).] Almost a month later, a one-day trial found Sasportas guilty of spying, punishable by death. Sasportas attempted to defend himself before the court, but Dubuisson chose to become a witness for the government, who spared his life in return for the damning testimony he provided.

Sasportas and the Subversive Geography of the Greater Caribbean

Sasportas's movements in the weeks and months prior to his arrest—in terms of places where we are able to situate him, his intended destinations,

---

[8] Sasportas to Louverture (October 2, 1799), C.O. 137/103, PRO.

and the areas that were to play a role in the attempt against Jamaica—map out a kind of subversive geography of the greater Caribbean. Charleston, for instance, had earlier in the decade been a major outfitting point for French privateers. Between 1793 and 1796, dozens of vessels under French colors cruised from Charleston to harass British and Spanish commerce, vessels whose owners and crews adopted names like *Le Vengeur* (The Avenger), *L'Ami de la Liberté* (The Friend of Liberty), *Le Vainqueuer de la Bastille* (The Conqueror of the Bastille), *L'Egalité*, *La Révolution*, *Le Sans-Culotte*, and even *La Guillotine*.[9] Further south, the diverse people who frequented St. Thomas exhibited various kinds of boundary-crossing that Sasportas would have appreciated. The shifting crews aboard the St. Thomas schooner, *Speedwell*, seized by a British cruiser while attempting to return to the Danish island from Saint-Domingue in 1793, reflected something of the character of this free port where Sasportas claimed to have business. The French crew that brought the *Speedwell* home from Saint-Dominigue was replaced by a St. Thomas crew in order to return. The latter group was in turn discharged in Jérémie in favor of a third crew consisting of "black free Men who could speak English." This crew, navigating the vessel at the time of its capture, were natives of Curaçao, except for one Michael Brown, a Barbadian who made his home on the Dutch island.[10]

Sasportas was very familiar with Curaçao, a place that had developed over the years a deserved reputation as a haven for troublemakers, particularly for fugitives fleeing Spanish justice. Organizers of an abortive 1797 conspiracy in Venezuela had recently escaped to Curaçao, which (in league with the radical French consul Jean-Baptiste Tierce) they used as a base for further efforts to spark an insurrection against Spanish authority in the sprawling and vulnerable Caracas captaincy general. Sasportas, on familiar terms with Tierce as well as some of the Spanish republicans, made a dramatic appearance in Curaçao in the summer of 1799, just months before his arrest. Styling himself as an official representative of the French Republic, Sasportas spoke uninhibitedly about the coming attempt on Jamaica, and

---

[9] See Melvin Jackson, *Privateers in Charleston, 1793–1796: An Account of a French Palatinate in South Carolina*. Washington, D.C.: Smithsonian Institution Press, 1969, p. 125.

[10] Examination of Michael Brown, n.d., in papers of the *Speedwell* (1793), JHCVA Papers, JA.

Dutch officials had him deported after he was implicated in a similar local conspiracy to establish French control in Curaçao.[11]

Sasportas arrived in Jamaica aboard a small Spanish vessel from Santiago de Cuba, where he claimed to have maintained a residence. Dubuisson, who met up with Sasportas there, complained to Roume that this "giddy Youth" lacked discretion, gambling for high stakes and once again making ill-considered and provocative public statements about what was about to happen in Jamaica.[12] Santiago de Cuba, too, was a site where a person of Sasportas's disposition and politics would have felt comfortable. A center for the landing of contraband and for illicit trade relations with Jamaica and Saint-Domingue, the eastern province's oversized jurisdictions, their residents scattered about the countryside and engaged mostly in small-scale farming, afforded "abundant opportunity," explained an official report in 1795, for wandering "idlers and vagabonds" to engage in all manner of mischief. Despite recent efforts of the governor in Havana to control this masterless population, their numbers had multiplied during the 1790s. Together with thousands of refugees from the French Caribbean, inhabitants of the city of Santiago de Cuba and its surrounding hinterlands made up a receptive audience, officials maintained, for the misguided notions of equality associated with the revolutions in France and neighboring Saint-Domingue.[13]

Port Antonio, Jamaica, the place where the French troops from Saint-Dominigue were to disembark, likewise represented a place of imperial exposure. As Jamaica's "North side" developed in the 18th century, Port Antonio and the other northern ports served as outlets to the sea for the island's most productive sugar-producing parishes: Hanover, St. James, Trelawny, St. Ann,

---

[11] See Antonio López Quintana to Miguel Cayetano Solér, September 3, 1800, Archivo General de Indias (hereafter AGI), Caracas, leg. 515; Isaac S. Emmanuel and Suzanne A. Emmanuel, *History of the Jews of the Netherlands Antilles*, 2 vols. (Cincinnati: American Jewish Archivist, 1970), 1:284–5; and Roberto Maria Tisnes J., *Movimentos pre-independientes Grancolombianos* (Bogotá: Academia Colombiana de Historia, 1963), 254–7.

[12] "Proceedings, ff 12, C.O. 137/103, PRO.

[13] Juan Baptista Vaillant to Luis de las Casas and enclosures, October 6, 1795, AGI, Papeles de Cuba, leg. 1435. For an extended discussion of the governor's efforts to contain "idlers and vagabonds," see Las Casas to Eugenio L'aguno and the enclosed *relación*, February 6, 1795, AGI, Santo Domingo, leg. 1263. For a general discussion of the Oriente district, see Eduardo Torres-Cuevas and Eusebio Reyes, *Esclavitud y Sociedad: Notas y documentos para la historia de la esclavitud Negra en Cuba* (La Habana: Editorial de Ciencias Sociales, 1986), 77–8.

St. Mary, and Portland. At the same time, these cities, situated close to foreign colonies and surrounded by "numerous creeks and bays, where small-decked vessels may run in at any time," provided staging areas for Jamaica-based smugglers and ports of call for their counterparts (like Sasportas) from Cuba, Saint-Dominigue, and elsewhere. When officials in Kingston and Spanish Town spoke about the north coast of the island, they always stressed the region's vulnerability. Defenseless against "the frequent Depredations made by the Spanish Boats from Cuba," residents of the northern ports also lived under the long shadow of "cockpit country" and the maroon towns. For all these reasons, reported Lieutenant Governor Adam Williamson discerningly in 1792, "the Spirit of discontent had usually first shewn itself" among Black residents of the north coast.[14]

Three years later, in 1795, Williamson's observations proved prescient, as north coast maroons staged an armed uprising, followed by a second attempt in 1798 (Figure 6.1). These chapters in the history of Caribbean resistance affected profoundly both Sasportas's developing politics and the strategic calculations of French officials in Saint-Domingue. Sasportas referred repeatedly to the important role that "Blue Mountain" insurgents would play in the coming Jamaican insurrection. In his lengthy report to Toussaint Louverture, he assured the military commander that he would make contact with maroon leaders. The "enormous cruelty" of the British had forced the maroons in 1795 to "raise the standard of revolt," Sasportas asserted. In 1799, however, they were "still oppressed and only awaiting the opportunity to recommence the struggle for their rights," an opportunity presented by the French plan. The remarkable, detailed working knowledge of this area of Jamaica reflected in Sasportas's report added some measure of legitimacy to his rhetorical flourishes. Road conditions, distances, and quite specific readings of the populations and the political state of major maroon towns provide one of the most impressive sections of this extraordinary document.[15]

---

[14] Jamaica Assembly, *Proceeding of the Honourable House of Assembly of Jamaica, on the Sugar and Slave Trade*, in a session which began the 23rd of October, 1792 (London: Stephen Fuller, 1793), 13; Philip Affleck to Philip Stephens, June 7, 1790, ADM 1/244, PRO; Adam Williamson to Henry Dundas, August 5, 1792, C.O. 137/90, PRO.

[15] Sasportas to Toussaint Louverture, October 2, 1799, C.O. 137/103, PRO.

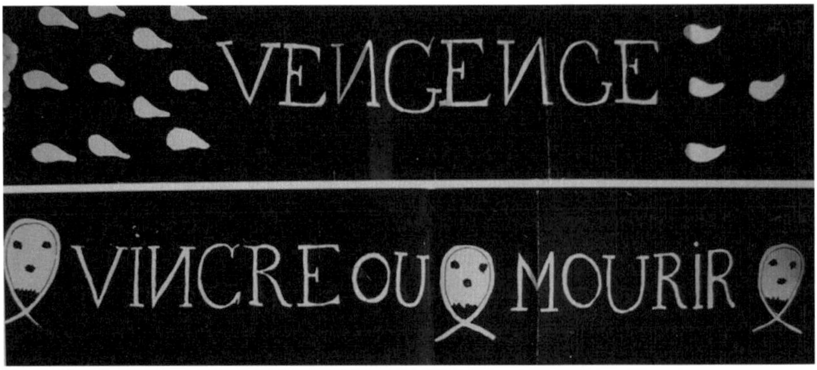

Figure 6.1. Sketch of French silk and silver strands armbands to be worn by slave rebels in the planned 1799 invasion of Jamaica. Enclosed in Balcarres to Portland (January 1, 1800), CO 137/103, British National Archives, Kew; photographed by Philippe R. Girard.

African and Jewish Caribbean Diasporas

Isaac Sasportas's deep immersion in the revolutionary currents of the Caribbean obviously raises larger questions about the nature of day-to-day relationships forged between Jews and Africans in Atlantic slave societies. By the late 18th century, those relationships had become part of an interesting discourse focused on issues of liberation and social transformation that involved both groups. First published in 1789, the ex-slave Olaudah Equiano's narrative of his life was among the first texts that explicitly articulated what he called "the strong analogy, which...appears to prevail in the early recognition of the affinity between African and Jewish diasporas."[16] Equiano stressed particular rites—circumcision, naming practices—and drew parallels between residents of his Ibo village of origin and the Jews described in the Old Testament. But one senses a West Indian origin in this framework as well, especially since Equiano himself worked as an enslaved seaman and much of his worldview evolved as a result of his experience in the maritime sector in which Caribbean Jews played pivotal roles. New World Jewry was Caribbean in origin. Some Jews were present in the West Indies as early as the 16th century, but they began to arrive in significant numbers as the Caribbean

[16] Olaudah Equiano, *The Interesting Narrative of the Life of Olaudah Equiano, or Gustavus Vassa, the African, Written by Himself*, new ed. (Leeds: James Nichols; London: Cradock and Joy; Darlington: W.H. Blackburn, 1814), reprinted in *The Classic Slave Narratives*, ed. Henry Louis Gates, Jr. (New York and London: Penguin, 1987), 20, 22–3.

moved away, beginning in the 1620s, from being a "Spanish lake" toward its new identity as a crossroads of empire and a site of cultural intermingling. Sephardic Jews from Brazil and Amsterdam began to settle in the newly established Dutch colony of Curaçao, whose first governor was a Dutch Jew, in the 1650s, establishing the first congregation there in 1654. From Curaçao, small contingents of Jews emigrated to Surinam, to Barbados, to Jamaica, and other territories, putting together in the process an increasingly elaborate commercial network that among other things linked the colonies of northern and western Europeans to markets in Spanish America.

By the 18th century, small but significant numbers of Jews could be found living and working in the islands and shorelines throughout the Caribbean.[17] To varying degrees, they were denied rights of citizenship everywhere. In Jamaica, for instance, laws passed during the 17th century denying Jews the right to hold public office, to vote in elections, to sit on juries, and to employ white servants remained in force through the early 1800s, and yet they could own property and even hold public worship. "They understood trade better than any of the planters or merchants could pretend to do," wrote the Jamaican historian Charles Leslie in 1740, so that "the Governor found it necessary to encourage" their presence in the British island. Similar concerns of tight restriction and the occasional begrudged concession characterized relations between Jews and colonial governments in other territories.[18]

Most 18th-century Jamaican Jews resided in the colonial capital of Spanish Town, where a Sephardi synagogue was erected in 1704 (the oldest in Britain's overseas empire), and an Ashkenazi synagogue was established just three years before Sasportas's execution. Contemporary writers vacillated, sometimes emphasizing the "industry and moderation" of the island's Jewish residents, at other times von Humboldt was finding them "roguish" and "tricky."[19] An account of an episode of military desertion from 1792 provides one suggestive example of some of the ways in which the latter framework regarding the Jewish presence in Jamaica could surface in particular instances of

---

[17] Throughout this period, the Jewish community in Curaçao remained the largest of any in the Caribbean—but even at its largest, the population of Jewish residents in the Dutch island only reached 2,000. See Seymour B. Liebman, *New World Jewry, 1493–1825: Requiem for the Forgotten* (New York: Ktav Publishing House, 1982), 169–191.

[18] Leslie is quoted in Benjamin Schlesinger, "The Jews of Jamaica: A historical view," *Caribbean Quarterly* 13 (March 1967), 47–48.

[19] See Schlesinger, "Jews of Jamaica," 48.

resistance. When, in February 1792, a group of ten musicians absconded from the 10th Regiment and headed for Kingston, they found shelter at the home of "a man of color," whose name was Jacob Hyam. Authorities arrested three of the deserters at Hyam's home; the rest escaped, and Hyam was sent to the parish jail. Magistrates tracked down all but two of the remaining deserters, an Irishman named George Theodorus Eskirkin and John Sims, a native of Quebec, within a couple of weeks. Eskirkin and Sims managed to stay on the lam with the aid of another notorious musician, "a black man named Jack Nailor," like Sims "a fiddler" who made his home in the area of Spanish Town known as "the Jew market." By mid-summer, exasperated authorities reported that Sims and Eskirkin had so effectively integrated themselves into Jamaica's teeming underground that they had become virtually indistinguishable from darker-skinned companions in Kingston and Spanish Town. Said to be "fishing and shooting" along the island's southern coast, the two musicians had come "to look as brown as some people of colour." There is no record of their having been taken up and returned to military duty.[20]

Evidence from several sources place other Caribbean Jews both inside and outside Saint-Domingue in positions by which they had something at stake in Saint-Domingue's struggle. Jewish residents of the colony, for instance, voiced opposition to the efforts of France's enemies to annex areas of Saint-Domingue. After Spanish forces invaded and occupied the small northern port of Fort Dauphin in the spring of 1794, they rounded up hundreds of fractious and troublesome local folk engaged in organizing opposition to Spanish authority. Topping a list of a diverse assortment of 110 "rabid republicans" and "denouncers of all Royalists" taken up in April and shipped off to Havana for confinement were the infamous Flores brothers, Luis and Rafael, whom officials described as "Jews who have vowed to re-establish the Republic" after engineering the ouster of the Spanish.[21]

Commerce between Saint-Domingue and other territories in the greater Caribbean—territories that Isaac Sasportas knew well—offered opportunities for Jewish residents of those areas to become involved in the revolution and to form some interesting alliances with individuals whose lives reflected the kind of boundary-crossing characteristic of the Jamaican conspirator.

---

[20] Kingston *Royal Gazette*, March 24, 31; May 5; June 22, 1792.

[21] See the *relación* enclosed with Luis de las Casas to Ministro de Guerra, La Habana, July 17, 1794, AGI, Papeles de Cuba, leg. 1488.

The activity of the St. Thomas vessel, *Trimmer*, captured leaving Les Cayes on Saint-Domingue's southern coast in March 1796, provides one example. Owned by the Jewish firm of Levy and Gomes in the Danish island, the *Trimmer* made repeated voyages to Saint-Domingue loaded with dry goods, wine, and other commodities. At the time of its capture, the Spanish schooner was under the command of a longtime acquaintance of the owners, ship's master Nicolas Manuel, a Spanish-speaking, Afro-Curaçaolien, naturalized burgher of St. Thomas, with an all-Black crew.[22]

Les Cayes was also the residence of Joseph and Donato Nathan, proprietors of a small commercial house during the 1790s. The Nathans acted as agents for the prominent Jewish merchant Moses Myers of Norfolk, Virginia, who owned several vessels that traded regularly between that port city and southern Saint-Domingue. By the spring of 1793, the Nathans had established themselves as merchants in Les Cayes, where they handled Myers's business along the southern coast of Saint-Domingue. By the mid-1790s, Les Cayes had become the most active port in the region in sponsoring, outfitting, and harboring French privateers. A Spanish visitor to Les Cayes in 1795 reported that more than thirty corsairs operated out of that port alone.[23] The Nathans apparently became well-connected participants in the emerging "republic" in and around Les Cayes. Citing "the zeal they have manifested in the Service of the French Republic," André Rigaud, the mulatto commander of French forces in the southern district, wrote in a letter to Moses Myers that the Nathans had earned "the esteem of all French Republicans in this place, the confidence of administration, and friendship."[24] The inspired language of Donato Nathan, as well as some of the activities in which the Nathans had begun to engage by this time, suggest why Rigaud valued their presence in Les Cayes. Surveying the situation in the Caribbean early in 1796, Donato Nathan expressed his excitement in terms that prefigured Sasportas's conspiracy. "The Tree of Liberty has taken root," he reported in a letter to Myers, and "all the Georges and Pitts in the universe will not change it, its beautiful Branches are already begin [sic] to spread over Jamaica." Nathan related with satisfaction the recent arrival of

[22] Examinations of Nicholas Manuel, March 26, May 3, 1796, papers of the *Trimmer* (1796), JHCVA Papers, JA.

[23] See the *relación* of Joaquin Garcia Jobe, with Quintana to Diego de Gardoqui, Caracas, June 30, 1795, AGI, Caracas, leg. 514.

[24] André Rigaud to Moses Myers, 1 Nivose, year 4 (December 22, 1795), in papers of Paragon (1796), JHCVA Papers, JA.

more than 400 British prisoners of war who had been captured in the eastern Caribbean by privateers loyal to Victor Hughes, the French commander at Guadeloupe, and were to be returned to Jamaica as part of a prisoner exchange. "You would have laughed," Nathan told Myers, "to hear those once brave soldiers Damned [sic] their King & Country on their landing, Many of them wishing to serve under the cap of liberty." The Nathans informed Myers that they had bought an American sloop "employed in trading from Port to Port," but in fact the ship they owned was a French privateer, whose real mission was "to hound the enemies of the French Republic" off the southern coast of Cuba—operating out of Santiago, Sasportas's ostensible place of residence.[25]

Jews in the Early 1800s in Colombia

Alexander von Humboldt, the German naturalist who visited Spanish America on a scientific expedition between 1799 and 1804, provides a fitting epilogue to this consideration of the range of Jewish involvement in the commercial and political networks tied to the French and Saint-Domingue revolutions.

Humboldt and his party arrived in Cartagena in the spring of 1801, just in time for Holy Week. They witnessed a series of elaborate rituals that reenacted familiar scenes from the last days in the life of Christ. Mendicants wearing crowns of thorns wandered from house to house, "with crucifix(es) in hand," begging alms. Plays based on biblical accounts were performed, one believer acting out the part of Pontius Pilate, others, as the twelve disciples, restaging the Last Supper. Some aspects of the celebration that year, however, appeared to relate more closely to tensions of the particular historical moment.

In Cuba and in Caracas, Humboldt had earlier noted evidence of the impact in Spain's colonies of the revolution in Saint-Domingue, and Cartegena's Caribbean location had linked that city to currents of rebellion in this quarter of the Atlantic world. Two years before Humboldt's visit, in May 1799 (about the time that Isaac Sasportas first established

[25] [Donato Nathan] to Moses Myers, January 21, 1796, in papers of Paragon (1796), JHCVA Papers, JA; André Rigaud to "Gobernador de la Ysla de Cuba en Santiago" (March 23, 1796), reprinted in *Documentos para la historia de Haiti en el Archivo Nacional,* ed. José Luciano Franco (La Habana: Publicaciones del Archivo Nacional de Cuba, 1954), 107–8.

contact with Charles), a number of recently arrived French-speaking slaves in Cartagena with ties to Saint-Domingue had conspired to take the city—in much the same way as Black rebels had taken Cap Français in 1793. In neighboring Turbaco, Humboldt would share lodgings with a group of French soldiers recovering from the costly attempt to reconquer Saint-Domingue for the Directory and he participated in "interminable discussions of the necessary cruelties that had been exercised against the Blacks of Saint-Domingue" in the course of that effort.

Increasingly attuned to the reverberations of the French Revolution in America as his trip unfolded, Humboldt recorded one particular Holy Week ritual, a "barbarous spectacle" that added a new twist. At sundown on Easter Sunday, several effigies meant to represent "Jews, dressed up in the French manner," appeared suspended from lampposts along the main streets in the city, their bodies "stuffed with straw and fireworks." The city's residents, related Humboldt, gathered excitedly to wait for the moment when "the Jews would be burned," their bodies exploding in a burst of light and sound. Townspeople were disappointed this year, Humboldt noted dryly, since unseasonable high humidity caused the French Jews to burn with less compelling effect than previous years.[26]

This symbolic execution, ritualized like Isaac Sasportas's hanging in Jamaica just a year-and-a-half earlier, made a more explicit, disturbing, and generalized reference to Jews as partisans in the Atlantic revolutions of the 1790s. What precisely to make of all this, scattered as the evidence is in bits and pieces across the entire region, much of it difficult to interpret, presents some interesting challenges. But what does seem clear is that the roles that Jews played in the Atlantic revolutions of the late 18th century, particularly in the Caribbean, merit closer attention, and that this important work challenges us to cross boundaries in much the same way as Sasportas managed to do in his short life.

---

[26] Alexander von Humboldt, *Relation historique dur voyage aux régions équinoxiales du Nouveau Continent*, 3 vols. (Stuttgart: F.A. Brockhaus, 1970), 3:558. For accounts of the Cartagena conspiracy of 1799, see Allan J. Kuethe, *Military Reform and Society in New Grenada, 1773–1808* (Gainesville: University Presses of Florida, 1978), 179, and Nicholás Castillo Mathieu, *Los gobernadores de Cartegena de Indias (1504–1810)* (Bogotá: Academia Colombiana de Historia, 1998), 122.

The Common Wind and Sasportas

Racism and anti-Semitism are often connected concepts historically, although the specifics of the treatment and relations of Blacks and Jews varied in different times and places. Blacks came to the Caribbean in the early 1500s on slave ships from Africa and Jews came in the 1490s fleeing from the Spanish Inquisition in Portugal and Spain. While very few Jews were plantation owners, some—such as Sasportas's uncle—did own slaves, and as merchants, they benefited from trade in slave-produced goods. An examination of precisely how relations between Jews and Blacks reflected connections between the ideals supported by the French and Haitian Revolutions and slavery practices in the Caribbean and the United States underscored Julius's interest in how "particular areas of the world connected to each other." As Julius explained to Nathan Connolly:

> The North American British colonies were part of a subregion that also included other places that people connected to. Ships from Philadelphia and Norfolk, for example, were all the time in different areas of the Caribbean. And those vessels, people, and the ideas they carried were connected to one another. That's what I wanted to try to get people to understand.

In his research which resulted in *The Common Wind*, he focused on connections among Black people:

> I wanted to know what one could say about the connections among Black people, about that particular relationship, to make Black people understood. There were some particularly important things to understand about the connection between people in South Carolina and people in Barbados, for example. You couldn't really understand the history of South Carolina without understanding how it was connected to Barbados…and the ways they tied into other places connected to them.
>
> [And] were there ways [that] Black North Americans connected to places and things that were outside of the world we thought they were in? What would be an 18th-century North American Black person's possibility to ever become aware that there was a Jamaica, or that there were British areas or Spanish areas? This became an important thing for me to understand. Could I find connected individuals who occupied different areas of the world at the same time, or who

> were moving from place to place, and were moving from parts of the Spanish world to parts of the English-speaking world, specifically?[27]

In his paper discussing the context of Isaac Sasportas's attempt to bring about a slave revolt in Jamaica, Julius sought to underscore how the Jewish merchants in the Caribbean were "individuals who occupied different areas of the world at the same time, or who were moving from place to place." Sasportas, while born in Cap Français in Saint-Domingue, also lived in Charleston, South Carolina; in Kingston, Jamaica; and in Santiago de Cuba and he continually traveled throughout the Caribbean as part of his trading business. His widespread connections and communications enabled him to devise the plan to begin a slave revolt in Jamaica, although as Julius notes, the plan was discovered by the British and Sasportas was subsequently executed.

It is unclear how representative Isaac Sasportas was in terms of Jewish support of abolition and the ending of slavery in the Caribbean in the late 18th century. The idea that Jews, like free-born Blacks, were not treated as legal citizens in Saint-Domingue (prior to the 1791 revolt), in Jamaica, and elsewhere supported Sasportas's view that race and religion had no place in the world of freedom, equality, fraternity to all. Yet while his uncle, Abraham, was also an advocate of the French and American revolutions, his ownership of slaves and his business interests reflected his ambivalent position. As Julius notes, "What precisely to make of all this, scattered as the evidence is in bits and pieces across the entire region, much of it difficult to interpret, presents some interesting challenges."

The literature on the history of Jews in the Caribbean, with some exceptions, does not consider in detail the extent to which Jewish merchants owned slaves. In the book, *Before Haiti: Race and Citizenship in French Saint-Domingue*, John Garragus (2006: 121–22) documents Jewish slave-owners in Saint-Domingue and discusses the situation of members of the prominent Jewish family, headed by Lopez Depas, who lived in the southern peninsula of Saint-Domingue. While subject to essentially anti-Semitic penalties by Charles Henri d'Estaing (Governor-general of Saint-Domingue and the Windward Islands from 1764 to 1766), several Depas family members had plantations and many slaves. It is unlikely that any of the Depas family

[27] From Interview, March 21, 2021, by Nathan Connolly, published in *Public Books*, 2022.

supported slave revolts or the abolition of slavery. After all, Isaac Sasportas's uncle owned slaves and did not support his nephew when sentenced:

> No member of Sasportas's family stepped forward publicly to defend his name, not even his radical uncle. Being associated with a slave conspiracy was evidently not good for business and could even be dangerous for members of a religious minority (Girard 2020: 431).

Indeed, with the exception of Isaac Sasportas, "none of [the Sasportas family]…went as far as advocating the abolition of slavery" (Girard 2020: 434). However, there were other Jewish families in the Caribbean and United States who were opposed to slavery and who saw, like Isaac Sasportas, the importance of freedom and equality for all, regardless of religion or race.

Conclusion

In his paper on Sasportas and the foiled attempt to launch a slave revolt in Jamaica, Julius referred to Alexander von Humboldt's visit to Cartagena during the Holy Week of 1801. He mentions that "a number of recently arrived French-speaking slaves in Cartagena with ties to Saint-Domingue had conspired to take the city—in much the same way as Black rebels had taken Cap Français in 1793." He also noted that the revolution in Saint-Domingue was related to French Jews' participation in the equally suspect French Revolution—at least from a Spanish perspective. The effigies of Jews, "dressed in the French manner," which were burned, suggests the complicated connections between slave revolts and slave ownership, racism and anti-Semitism, and Jews in the Atlantic world, connections which have infrequently been studied.

Chapter 7
On Race

Julius taught several undergraduate classes, including Dynamics of the Black Diaspora (CAAS 211) and Survey of Afroamerican History (CAAS 230, History 274), that examined the issue of race in various settings. As Julius noted in a PowerPoint presentation on race in November 2015, race is a complicated concept. In his first slide, he listed several different perspectives on the meaning of the word, race:

- Race—its relationship to slavery and its aftermath(s) in the Americas
- Blackness/Brownness/Whiteness ("three-tiered racial order")
- Race across boundaries—comparative approach/focus on how things circulate
- Race as biological/social category ("socially constructed")

As a historian, he was interested in how these different categorizations of race played out in different times and in different places. The courses that he taught at the University of Michigan (UM) exemplify this perspective.

One book that he discussed in his classes was *Slavery Disowned: Gradual Emancipation and "Race" in New England, 1780–1860*, by Joanne Melish, who discusses a particular view of "race," represented in government documents, New England town records, newspaper articles, antebellum Black literature, as well as historical society and library collections. While New England states abolished slavery in the late 18th century, long before the civil war, attitudes toward Black people reflected an "uneasy juxtaposition of advocacy and aversion, of desire for justice (or, at least, desire to evade complicity in injustice) and longing for erasure that characterized a broad range of antislavery thinking in its abolitionist, colonizationist, and nativist manifestations in antebellum New England" (Melish 1998: xiii). The discourse of slavery had been transformed into the discourse of "race." Hence, "race" came to be thought of as a set of characteristics—with people of the White "race" as competent, independent, and reliable, while people of the Black "race" whose incapacity, dependency, and need for external control made them inferior even once they were freed from slavery.

Another way of thinking about race, as Julius explained, had to do with shades of skin color and how they aligned with social and political hierarchy. He utilized the recordings of the Trinidadian calypso singer, Lord Kitchener, that expressed this situation. Thus, the song, "If You're Brown" speaks to a system of racial thinking that has three tiers—black, brown, white ("If you're white, you're right. If you're brown, hang around. If you're black, get back;" Lord Kitchener 2004).

Julius brought his research on Caribbean and US history into the discussion of race across boundaries—taking a comparative approach for thinking about how ideas about slavery and race circulate. For example, the Haitian 1805 Constitution defines all citizens as "Black," whereas in South Carolina, one was considered Black with one drop of Black blood while only white-skinned people with no Black ancestors were considered White.

Julius also introduced students to the idea that race was a "socially constructed" category, as a form of ethnicity that reflected place of origin, history, language, as well as skin color. This approach differs from the thinking of Leland Stanford, the co-founder of Stanford University:

> I am in favor of free white American citizens. I prefer free white citizens to any other class or race. I prefer the white man to the negro as an inhabitant of our country. I believe its greatest good had been derived by having all of the country settled by free white men (Riskin 2023: 34).

However, current anthropology textbooks have qualified the use of the term, race, in favor of ethnicity: Skin color may be one of the qualities on which ethnic identity is based, but the genetic basis of skin color is variable—there is not one gene that uniformly determines skin color and hence "race." Thus, race has been defined as "an ethnic group assumed to have a biological basis," assumed, not biologically determined, while ethnicity is the preferred term to distinguish individuals identifying with, and feeling part of, and distinct from other social groups.

These distinctive discussions of the concept of "race" could be, at times, difficult to teach:

> Julius was so bummed out about his mostly (White male) students, refusing to accept his argument about the English Americans, about the English demographic decline, that somehow their ideas about early Americans are rooted in the idea that the country was English, in other words, White (Journal, January 27, 2009).

On Black History Month

However, the shared histories of slavery, of racial discrimination, of linguistic slurs, among other insults to their humanity, led to Black historians underscoring the importance of the achievements of Black Americans. Initially, there was Negro History Week, initiated in 1926, by Dr. Carter Woodson, the second African American to receive a PhD in history from Harvard University, and Reverend Jesse Moorland, founders of the Association for the Study of Negro Life and History (ASNLH). They sought to bring about a focus in schools and churches on the history of African Americans and to emphasize the Black contributions to US society. This week was later extended to Black History Month, informally in the late 1960s on several college campuses, and officially by President Gerald Ford, in 1976.

In 1991, Julius was interviewed by Dr. Caroline Lattimore at Duke University. The focus of their discussion was Black History Month and why it continues to be important for Black people in the United States. As Julius observed: "For Black people, looking upon our history goes beyond the history itself but rather serves as an inspiration for the direction we'd like to move. We need to go back to the well-spring to understand ourselves."

Dr. Lattimore then asked Julius to explain the history of Black History Month and he referenced the efforts of Professor Carter G. Woodson (Woodson 1922). Indeed, along with Woodson's work, Julius noted that Negro History Week "has expanded because teachers, students, and clergy have thought of Black history as being so important... For we all have to make sure that America begins to recognize the diversity of people's backgrounds."

> Dr. Woodson, as the Father of Negro History, had two objectives, one external and one internal. For the external objective, he wanted to speak to the culture at large. We Blacks have really contributed, we have been an integral part of this nation from its founding—you can't understand the United States unless you understand the contributions of African Americans as being central to that purpose. This was said in the 1920s and 1930s. However, his internal purpose, when talking to Blacks themselves was that by knowing that, we are to demand the rights we deserve and strive to stand up for Black agency and to demand from White Americans the recognition of African Americans in US history (Lattimore 1991. Interview: Julius Scott, 1991, Durham, North Carolina).

Both Julius and Dr. Lattimore agreed that standing up for Black rights was as important in 1991 as it was in 1926. One could add that it continues to be important in 2023.

Education and Race

As has been discussed in Chapter 3, Julius was one of the first African American students to attend MacGregor Primary School in Houston, Texas, in 1961. When his family moved to Providence, Rhode Island, he attended an integrated primary school, and later, when they moved again, to Atlanta, Georgia, he attended an all-Black primary school there. However, his father wanted him to attend the newly integrated private secondary school, Westminster Academy, which has a long history of segregation and racism. For example, Julius told a group at a UM faculty dinner about the Slave Day fundraiser (Journal, December 19, 2019). This event has been described in an *Atlanta Journal-Constitution* account:

> The first black students at Westminster encountered blatant racism and jarring celebrations of the south's racist past, including an annual fundraiser patterned after a "slave" auction and a junior-senior Old South ball in which students were told, "the foyer and front lawn will be decorated as a southern plantation…gentlemen may wear either old Confederate uniforms or tuxedos" (Downey 2019).

Slave Day was also discussed in a volume on the desegregation of private schools in the South, with a specific discussion of Westminster Academy:

> In January 1956, "Slave Market Provides Rat's Revenge on Seniors," one can see how students discussed the slave auction, an annual fundraiser for the Atlanta Child's Home. One description of the auction involved the sons of Ivan and Louise Allen Jr. The reporter wrote, "Ivan Allen became the unworthy slave of Inman [Allen] who had as his assistant John Mullin, Jimmy Fluker, and Tommy Rains. Ivan started off Wednesday by crawling around the gymnasium floor and then serving Inman and Tommy a Coke just before Mr. Austin's English Class."… These racially charged pictures, depictions, and events at Westminster point to how Westminster embraced racist forms in the years before desegregation as a southern institution that attempted to provide a nationally recognized education. Based on how they conceptualized U.S. slave auctions of those of African descent, young men auctioned one another, and the event seemed popular among students, faculty, and staff. As this southern school would continue to develop, it would include a school culture that manifested values related to race (Purdy 2018: 44–45).

Julius mentioned how other members of the Westminster community had to adjust their behavior with the admission of Black students to the school:

> Julius told another story, this time about a friend who was on the football team, probably the first Black student the coach had had. The coach, Buck ****, used to use all sorts of racist language to talk to his team—"nigger," "slaves", etc. So he had to start reining it in with a Black student on the team. Julius said there were four Black male students at Westminster when he was there, and two Black women students at its sister school but then he left (Journal, April 24, 2011).

Julius was also personally affected, when as a freshman at Westminster, he was a popular candidate for class president, but he was not allowed to be elected to the office because he would have had to kiss the White class queen from Westminster's sister school (Journal, November 29, 1999).

Yet even with tacit integration, life in many ways did not change for African American students:

> Julius was talking about Westminster, how there were only two Black students in his class when he started and that one student left after his first year. Then Julius was the only one. The next year he went to Indian Springs School where there were four Black students. The way he put it, "when you'd go home, you'd

> be back in the Black community, regardless of school 'integration'" (Journal, September 19, 2012).

After leaving Westminster for Indian Springs School, he participated in many activities including the school choir and soccer. When playing in a soccer match at other private schools in Alabama, racist remarks were not uncommon, although he rarely had any negative experiences otherwise (Journal, December 3, 2019).

> Julius was so amusing at dinner, talking about his trips as part of the Indian Springs choir, staying with a Black family in Champaign, Illinois, who named their children after Greek politicians, classical scholars—Xerxes, etc., and listened to avant-garde jazz. Or the family that fed them cheesy ravioli or congratulating themselves when the *New York Times* referred to them as an integrated choir. And that they, the handful of Black students, were responsible for their claim (Journal, October 29, 2010).

He also told a story about his Indian Springs high school choir group trip that went to Kenosha, Wisconsin:

> The Black choir members were put up with Black families. The family they stayed with, the daughters were sick so their father went out to buy Kentucky Fried Chicken for his guests. When they got back and he opened the carton, there was cigar ash on the chicken. "Those dirty buzzards!" he said. They didn't eat the chicken (Journal, December 12, 2016).

After graduating from Indian Springs School, Julius attended Brown University where he was known as DJ, for Dr. Julius. (Dr. J was a reference to Julius Irving, the famous basketball player at the time.) And he had some Black classmates, some of whom he liked and some of whom he didn't:

> Julius told some hilarious stories about his classmates at Brown. One was a student nicknamed Pops for PK or popcorn who was a wacky wordsmith and really a poet. One of the students whom he didn't like (a political science/Russian major), also African American, he referred to as the Black Russian; there were other words that he used when he didn't like someone.

> Julius read *The Invisible Man* by Ralph Ellison and fell in love with it; he wrote a very detailed, deep paper that his (White) Brown professor didn't understand. Julius said he was very hurt (Journal, June 30, 2015).

Julius had a generally favorable experience of graduate school at Duke University where he conducted research for his PhD dissertation, *The Common Wind: Afro-American Currents in the Age of the Haitian Revolution*, which later became his award-winning book. He did mention, however, an incident that disturbed his White landlord and some of his Black friends:

> Julius told the story of one racist incident in his neighborhood in Durham, North Carolina, when people across the street put a (Black) jockey statue light on their front lawn. He said that he ignored it, but that his landlord (a young White man) made a disparaging remark about the statue and his neighbor. Julius said that some of his Black friends avoided coming to his house after the statue first appeared and he realized then that it was causing friction. One day soon after the statue appeared, people woke to see that it had a new face—a White face (Journal, June 27, 2013).

After attending Duke, he took up an assistant professor position briefly at the University of Illinois, Circle Campus, and then came back to Duke where he taught for six years, from 1988 to 1994. His discussion with Dr. Lattimore took place when he was there. In 1996, he went to New York University for a year and then to the University of Michigan, where he worked until he retired in 2018.

On Race Relations in Michigan

Judging from his comments about various experiences of his life in Michigan and his teaching at the University of Michigan, it was a racially ambiguous place. Parts of the state, especially urban centers such as Detroit and Flint, have majority Black populations while areas in the northern parts of the state are largely White. This divide is reflected in some White attitudes toward Detroit residents:

> The "caretaker" for Detroit [when the mayor was being investigated], in an interview in the *Wall Street Journal*, said that Detroit had long suffered from

> fat, lazy, careless use of wealth—a comment which brought a lot of criticism from (Black) residents. One man responded saying that he'd worked all his life and put money in his pension program, which has now disappeared. It was surprising that no one said the obvious—that these words/images have long been caricatures stereotyping Blacks in this country. "Don't they think of what they are saying?" Julius astutely answered, "They know exactly what they are saying." He's right, of course (Journal, August 6, 2013).

While Ann Arbor, Michigan, had a mainly White population, there were some Black, Latino/a, and Asian members of the community, which reflected its location as the home of the University of Michigan. Nonetheless, being a minority fostered careful behavior at times:

> Julius told an interesting story about when he went to vote (at Pittsfield Town Center). There were as usual relatively few Blacks. But unlike other elections when Black people greeted each other, this time they didn't. Julius thought it was because they didn't want White people to think it was some sort of cabal, Obama being elected by Blacks. Similarly, there was a *New York Times* story about Florida Blacks, walking on eggs, being on their "best behavior" so as not to jeopardize Obama's chances (Journal, November 5, 2008).

Generally, Julius went about his business, going to the university, to the grocery store, and to his apartment and later, house. However, it wasn't always easy to get by without incident. One afternoon he had a very unpleasant experience:

> Julius did a very funny rendition of appearing before Judge Judi about a police incident yesterday. Julius was sitting in his car [in his parking space at his apartment building], minding his own business and listening to sports radio and someone reported him to the police. He thinks it was a heavy-set, older White woman he'd seen living in a neighboring apartment. The police knocked on his window and asked to see his driver's license.
>
> So Julius's mock court scene was about harassment and racism. The defendant did a long complaint about all the robberies that the plaintiff was involved in, how he was sitting, waiting for her to go out. Julius was really upset, as if he doesn't have enough to be unhappy about (Journal, September 1, 2001).

This example of a White woman's accusation of a Black man reflected attitudes that led to voters' reassessment of Affirmative Action in Michigan, which had consequences for the University of Michigan.

Affirmative Action in Michigan

In April 2003, the US Supreme Court ruled on the question of whether a White applicant to the University of Michigan Law School could be denied admission based on the Law School's "compelling interest in achieving diversity among its student body." In a 5–4 decision the court ruled that use of race in considering student admissions did not violate the Equal Protection Clause of the Fourteenth Amendment or Title VI of the Civil Rights Act of 1964, "because the Law School conducts highly individualized review of each applicant, no acceptance or rejection is based automatically on a variable such as race and that this process ensures that all factors that may contribute to diversity are meaningfully considered alongside race."[1]

Yet three years later, on November 7, 2006, Michigan residents in a ballot initiative, known as Proposal 2, Affirmative Action Initiative, voted to end affirmation action based on "a state constitutional ban on race-conscious admissions" at Michigan universities, which included the University of Michigan. Subsequently, "Black undergraduate enrollment declined to 4 percent in 2021 from 7 percent in 2006, the brief said, even as the total percentage of college-age African Americans in Michigan increased to 19 percent from 16 percent" (Saul 2022). One possible consequence of this change occurred in April 2007, when:

> Someone (or persons) had gone through Haven Hall [where the Department of Afroamerican and African Studies is located], putting up signs saying "Whites only," "Coloured only" on the drinking fountains sometime around 9am. It was very creepy especially in light of Proposal 2 and the Virginia Tech shooting [on April 16, 2007]. But Julius was right to question the intentions of the sign distributors. It could have been BAM [Black Action Movement] students making a point about how Proposal 2 could lead to this separate race thing or create "helter-skelter" or it could be *Michigan Review* types [who supported

---

[1] Oyez 2003. *Grutter v. Bollinger*, https://www.oyez.org/cases/2002/02-241, accessed July 9, 2023.

> ending affirmative action]. It's not clear and Julius, being the sort of person he is, noticed that (Journal, April 19, 2007).

The signs were almost immediately taken down.

There were also less obviously offensive but nonetheless contradictory racial relations at the university. For example, the UM football team had Black and White players and their parents would often attend games to watch their sons in action. Julius was talking with a Black staff member about his son's outstanding performance and heard an additional part of the story:

> One staffer goes to UM football games when his son plays—and that the Black parents of players who go see him as their ambassador with the White parents of players—since neither group—Black and White—have much interaction with one another. Apparently, they don't feel comfortable or even like one another. As Julius said, "You might expect this in Mississippi, but this is Michigan. But it is essentially a very segregated state" (Journal, October 25, 2009).

Another interaction involving faculty assumptions about race and academic status was experienced by Julius himself:

> Julius said he ran into a White colleague in the elevator, talking with someone who'd come to hear a guest speaker. "XX, I don't know him either, but his department, I think it's history," which infuriated Julius. "It's just another way that the Department of Afroamerican and African Studies (DAAS), which has Black and White faculty, is dismissed when people assume that it wouldn't be possible for a prestigious White scholar, such as XX, to have a 100% appointment in DAAS, since it would imply that the person was in a 'light-weight' disciplinary department."
>
> Julius pointed out another way that Black-White gets played out by White faculty members. That another DAAS colleague [who was White] could, tongue-in-cheek, refer to DAAS as a "colorful" unit—but that Black faculty could never refer to it as an equally Black and White unit—a "salt and pepper" unit, that it would be considered impolite to point this out (Journal, September 17, 2009).

Despite the attitudes that such comments represented, Julius generally had a positive experience at the University of Michigan, both with his colleagues and his students. Indeed, his sense of humor helped him. Thus, he noted some of the things that his students said or did:

> Julius was funny last night, doing imitations of why students were taking CAAS 111. "My boyfriend's Black so I wanted to learn more about his culture." So he launched into a version of "My boyfriend's back"—"My boyfriend's Black and there's gonna be trouble…" (Journal, September 9, 2004).
>
> Julius was amusing this morning, doing a riff about students getting professors to explain things to them by flattery. He compared it to slaves getting the massa to show them how to hoe cotton. "I hoed the whole field to show those dumb Negroes how to do it…" (Journal, December 2, 2006).

He also observed the irony of a comment made by a donor at a UM library event:

> Julius told an interesting story about going to a UM Library lunch to honor the donor of some slave-ship owner's papers (the donor's ancestor), who said to Julius, "Well, we probably have more in common than anyone else here," since few other Black people were in attendance. Julius said he was thinking (to himself), "What, that you're a millionaire and I make $50,000?" (Journal, March 24, 2002).

On Race and Health Care

While reports of health care for Blacks in the US document racial discrimination, Julius rarely experienced openly racist behavior although some doctors' remarks implied it. Thus, one young doctor in Plastic Surgery told him, "You need to get your diabetes under control!" As if Julius had not been attending to his diabetes care for many years (Journal, May 7, 2015). Another incident was inadvertent:

> There was a very humorous complication, actually another one of the bizarre stories about his prosthesis. Julius had gotten a new prosthesis and they needed

> to put a foot on it. But they only had a white one, the black leg he had didn't match it. The prosthetist was incredibly apologetic (Journal, November 4, 1999).

It was hard to know precisely how his treatment at the University of Michigan Hospital was associated with race and how much was simply that he was such a frequent patient, that some things were bound to be prejudicial. He did like many of his doctors who treated him with kindness and dignity. He also had some pleasant interactions with some, but not all, fellow patients:

> The most wonderful part of the emergency room stay was when there was an elderly Black man in the next bed. After the man went to the bathroom, he and Julius greeted each other as he walked back to his bed. When the man left with his son, they both smiled at Julius and said good night (Journal, November 7, 1999).

Conclusion

Race is indeed a difficult subject to teach. One way that Julius sought to get his students to think about different meanings was by suggesting alternative uses of the "quote marks" regarding issues relating to race. Thus, he argued that the phrase, Disowning "Slavery," could refer to the ideological rather than literal meaning of the word, slavery, as discussed in the book, *Slavery Disowned*, mentioned in this chapter's introduction. The idea of slavery was abolished but in actuality, it continued to be practiced in various manifestations. Similarly, the phrase, "Emancipation" and Race, reflected the ideological meaning of emancipation, rather than its literal meaning, since African Americans continued to be relegated to demeaning work and discrimination in the Jim Crow South.

He considered the phrases "Gradual" Emancipation and Race, and Gradual "Emancipation" and Race in a similar way. As Joanne Melish (1998: 2) explains it in the case of New England, from 1780 to 1860:

> The process of gradual emancipation had mapped the old assumptions about slaves onto a new class of person, "free negro"; the old assumptions about the mutability of servile characteristics had been transformed into a new conviction of their innateness and immutability.

Both the words, gradual and emancipation, had ideological meanings but also literal meanings that belied what they appeared to mean, just as integration at Houston primary school did not literally mean desegregation of bathrooms for Black students as Julius himself experienced.

Teaching about race and how it is defined can also be risky. Thus, when the University of Chicago lecturer, Dr. Rebecca Journey, announced a new undergraduate anthropology course, entitled "The Problem of Whiteness," to be taught in 2023, she received numerous hostile emails. Even though the course was structured to consider the changing ways that the word, White, relating to race, has been defined, because of the controversy surrounding it, the course was ultimately postponed and eventually was not taught.

The tweet that was sent by a University of Chicago undergraduate student stated that "'Anti-white hatred is now mainstream academic inquiry,' along with the course description and Dr. Journey's photo and university email address" (Patel 2023). Julius's response might have been, "The arrogance of White people!" (Journal, January 26, 2003). That the issue of race as reflected in the recent Supreme Court decision concerning affirmative action has become increasingly volatile in the early 21st century suggests that arguments over the meaning of race continue to be a source of discord, disagreement, and discrimination in the United States.

Chapter 8

Memories and Memorials

Julius Scott passed away on the morning of December 6, 2021, just after midnight. He was unconscious, in a bed in the University of Michigan Hospital—alone because the Covid restrictions did not allow family members to stay overnight with him. But in a way, it was a quiet reprieve from all the medical interventions that he had suffered through—at last he was in peace.

The Covid pandemic and the dispersed locations of family and friends delayed the memorial service at St. Andrew By-the-Sea United Methodist Church in Hilton Head, SC, which was held on February 5, 2022. The service and program were organized by Ann (Ianthia Harrell) Scott, Julius's mother, and was well attended by many in the community and from out of town. Music included "Sidewinder" by Lee Morgan, "Dear Lord" by John Coltrane (along with a silent reading of the lyrics), and the hymn by Thelonious Monk, "Abide with Me." Sabrina Harrell, Julius's cousin, and David Scott, Julius's brother, read passages from the Holy Bible: the 23rd Psalm ("The Lord is my shepherd...") and Romans 5: 1–5, 10–11 ("Therefore, since we are justified by faith, we have peace with God..."). Reflections were offered by Julius's cousin, Deborah Feaster:

> Scotty was that rare pearl that left his mark on people everywhere, especially me. He was so calming in nature, and so full of wisdom. From my observation, while in his presence, he only spoke when he had something to say. (February 5, 2022, Hilton Head, SC)

And by Willard Brooks:

> I give all honor and praise to our ancestors who came before us and put in motion the circumstances that led to the life of our beloved cousin... Scotty was described by some of his cousins as: "Courageous and full of joy and humor,"

> "A quiet and intelligent observer," "A lovable person with a few words but a huge heart," and "A gentle, humble spirit, a genius without the arrogance."
>
> His groundbreaking book, *The Common Wind*...is a masterful piece of work as it lets us in on the secrets of our journeys throughout the Americas, but more importantly, it documents how, even under the most repressive circumstances, those in power could never extinguish the light of us by cutting off any means of our communication. As much as they tried, they could not hold back The Common Wind! (February 5, 2022, Hilton Head, SC)

Words of comfort were given by Lamar Scott, Julius's brother.

> As we reflect on Scotty's PURPOSE, in learning from him, we know we can take our intellect and continue to dream, and continue to strive for excellence. We know that we can enjoy each other NOW and the life around us regardless of our circumstances...and even laugh at life on occasion, while also persevering and remaining positive through life's many challenges. This was the way Scotty lived his life every day and it's through these things that we can honor him and continue his legacy. (February 5, 2022, Hilton Head, SC)

The service ended with a Benediction given by the officiating pastor, Dr. Robin Dease.

After the service, Julius's ashes were taken to Six Oaks Cemetery, in Hilton Head, and placed in a grave next to his father's.

Memories, Memorials

While the news of Julius's death did not surprise people who knew of his long struggle with diabetes, it did inspire many people to write about his life and his contributions to their own. The memories and memorials of friends, colleagues, doctors, students, and other family members were remarkable in their admiration for Julius as a person and of his work.

His cousin, Shaykh Muhammad Shareff, who lives in Mali, West Africa, sent a eulogy and prayers:

> In the name of GOD, the Beneficent the One whom there is nothing like Him
>
> And peace and blessings upon the one whom there will be no prophet after him

> To my cousin, the erudite historian, the professor, whom we all fondly called Scotty
>
> You now know that this world is fleeting with all of its allurements and empty folly
>
> Like the griots of ancient Mali, you've transcended death with your work *The Common Wind*
>
> You've brought to life our history and revived our story which our enemies tried hard to rescind
>
> The ancient sages say that when you successfully write the history of a people, you give life to them
>
> May GOD give life to you, Scotty, each time one recalls our struggle for freedom and liberation stratagem…
>
> May GOD the Exalted join you in the company of your learned father, whose honorable
>
> name and intelligence you share
>
> May He console your blessed mother, our aunt Nini; your siblings David, Lamar and all who had you under their care
>
> Like all your erudite colleagues and students who have taken you as their academic model and paradigm
>
> And all those who will one day read *The Common Wind* and rediscover our ongoing struggle for freedom in their lifetime
>
> Farewell, my cousin, until we meet again; may your erudition keep you company as you rest in eternal peace
>
> And inspire others in turn, as you did, to revive our African heritage and cause its indomitable values to increase. (February 4, 2022, Mali, West Africa)

Shaykh is looking forward to the French translation of *The Common Wind.*

Others, living in the United States and Canada, have written about their memories of Julius. One of his longtime friends wrote the following remembrance.

> Julius Scott, "Scotty," has been my dear friend since we met. We were of among twenty Black boys approaching ninth grade at an academic camp geared to prepare us for the rigors of private school. Everyone loved Scotty Scott. He was fun with an infectious smile and great sense of humor. Of course, he was super smart. He also punched above his weight on the playground.

At his high school, Indian Springs, he earned and enjoyed the same adoration and respect from everyone. I could also sense something else about him. He was becoming more of Julius than Scotty. More of Julius, on the pathway to becoming an esteemed scholar, like his Dad. Our cultural and American mantra is that you can be anything. Well, that sounds great but as we know sometimes reality kicks in and tempers dreams. Reality, more often than not, is in the form of limitations of ability or opportunity. Part of my admiration for Julius includes the awareness that this man could have truly been almost anything. I could easily envision him as a great research scientist or physician working cutting edge science to save lives. Or as a legal scholar and a judge worthy of Supreme Court consideration. The world of academia is indeed fortunate for his presence as an educator of young minds who would go forth and impact their worlds.

As I took in the deterioration of his condition, throughout it all, Julius projected the greatest display of dignity and resilience I have ever witnessed. I also witnessed a beautiful and powerful embodiment of love and devotion as he was blessed with. (February 5, 2022)

Tom Montgomery, Class of 1973, another close friend of Julius from the Indian Springs School, fondly remembered their time together.

I was saddened to hear of the death of Julius Sherrod "Scotty" Scott III, class of 1973, on December 6th of this year. Scotty was one of the most talented people I have ever met. He was bright, athletic, and a very good singer for the glee club. He was an all-American in soccer; maybe not so much in basketball as he was the happy recipient of the Arm Pitt award. But what I most remember him for is that he was very funny, a great mimic, and always friendly. All students and faculty treasured and enjoyed being around Scotty: Doc Armstrong; Mr. Fleming (not surprisingly Scotty majored in history at Brown and got his Ph.D. in history at Duke); Mr. Draper (unbeknownst to Mr. Draper is that Scotty could do a wicked-good imitation of him… "Scotty I haven't seen you at the French table lately"); coach Cameron; Joe Mays; Charles Ellis; Ms. Dearing; Mr. Jennings; Mr. Campbell; Mr. Stegner; Ms. Lake—the campus nurse; and Jack—the nightwatchman. Unbeknownst to Jack was that Scotty could do a pitch-perfect imitation of Jack… ("uh, what you boys doing in there?"). Everyone on campus knew and liked Scotty.

Scotty was one of the first African Americans admitted to Indian Springs, coming the year after Darrell Jones '73 and James Montgomery '73, and he was the first African American Mayor at Springs. Hard as it is to believe now, someone in the ISS [Indian Springs School] office called me before I went there as a 10th grader and asked if it would be okay if I had a Black suitemate. Of course, I said yes. That suitemate was Darrell Jones '73 and he and I became roommates our junior and senior years. Scotty was one of the "band of boarders" who spent most weekends on campus. Along with Darrell, Douglas Hunter '73, Jeff Humphries '73, Bruce Lilly '74, and others, we would stay up all night on the weekends talking about sports, our classes, and girls or the lack thereof.

After Indian Springs, Scotty went on to great success and was a respected and well-known historian. He was a long-standing tenured Professor of History at the University of Michigan where he wrote the highly-acclaimed book, *The Common Wind*, which is a ground-breaking account of the Haitian revolution and described how enslaved people formed underground communities throughout the Americas. And yet it is the memories of Scotty at Indian Springs that meant so much to so many: the encouragement and acceptance of everyone by Indian Springs as we strived to learn through living, congregating and laughing at our table in the dining hall, going to Europe with the Glee Club, the time Scotty scored a goal in the last minute up in Tennessee, the Derf rallies, and so many more.

Thank you, Scotty, for allowing all of us to spend some more time with you. May you now rest and be long remembered. (December 15, 2021)

After graduating from Indian Springs School, Julius studied history at Brown University and then went on to Duke University, where he became friends with a fellow history PhD student, Paul Krause. Paul recalls Julius and their aborted plan to meet again:

I have some sense of how rewarding it was to be with Julius, and also how difficult it could be, and I also know that his memory will be a blessing. I rarely post anything on Facebook, but I published the attached photo and the following blurb:

"Julius and I had planned a celebratory mini-reunion in Ann Arbor on the occasion of the publication of his book, but of course the pandemic intervened, and we could not carry out the plans to re-enact our graduate school pastimes

> of bourbon and high-jinks and gossip about the quirks of our beloved, truly beloved, faculty mentors at Duke. Julius was never so happy as when *The Common Wind* was published. Never. He was new and whole.
>
> Years and years ago, he came to Vancouver. My son, Ben, was just a little guy then, and for him reading and soccer were the world. He grabbed Julius's hand and led him to the breakfast table, and they read for a while together, and then Ben somehow discovered that Julius had played soccer at Brown. This led to a clinic of the beautiful game in the front yard: there they were, two perfectionists who knew instantly, intuitively, that this not-so-secret quality defined and bound them together.
>
> This is a photo of that day, and all of the gentleness and warmth in Julius is right there. He endured so much pain and loss, and I cannot recall a word of complaint or any sense of unfairness. This is what I am sure all who knew and loved him are feeling now."
>
> I would like to think that Julius did find a safe place to be sad. (December 8, 2021, Vancouver, British Columbia, Canada; Figure 8.1)

When he heard of Julius's passing, another good friend from Duke, Jim Leitzel, exclaimed "What a heavy blow. What a loss. So sorry about this sad, sad turn of events. Still hard to take it all in" (December 7, 2021, Chicago, Illinois). Jim had traveled to Hilton Head to observe the funeral for Julius's father whom he had also known for quite some time. One thing he didn't know was Julius's cap size:

> I recall that Scotty has a birthday on the horizon and I want to send him a baseball cap. But, of course, I don't know his size, and I am looking at non-adjustable caps. Any chance you know his cap size off-hand? (I do remember that his hats were always too big for me!) (July 31, 2018, Chicago, Illinois)

Faculty Friends and Colleagues

Paul Krause mentioned "the quirks of our beloved, truly beloved, faculty mentors at Duke." Peter Wood was one of the most truly beloved history faculty there, who mentored Julius and also got to know his parents, as he explained.

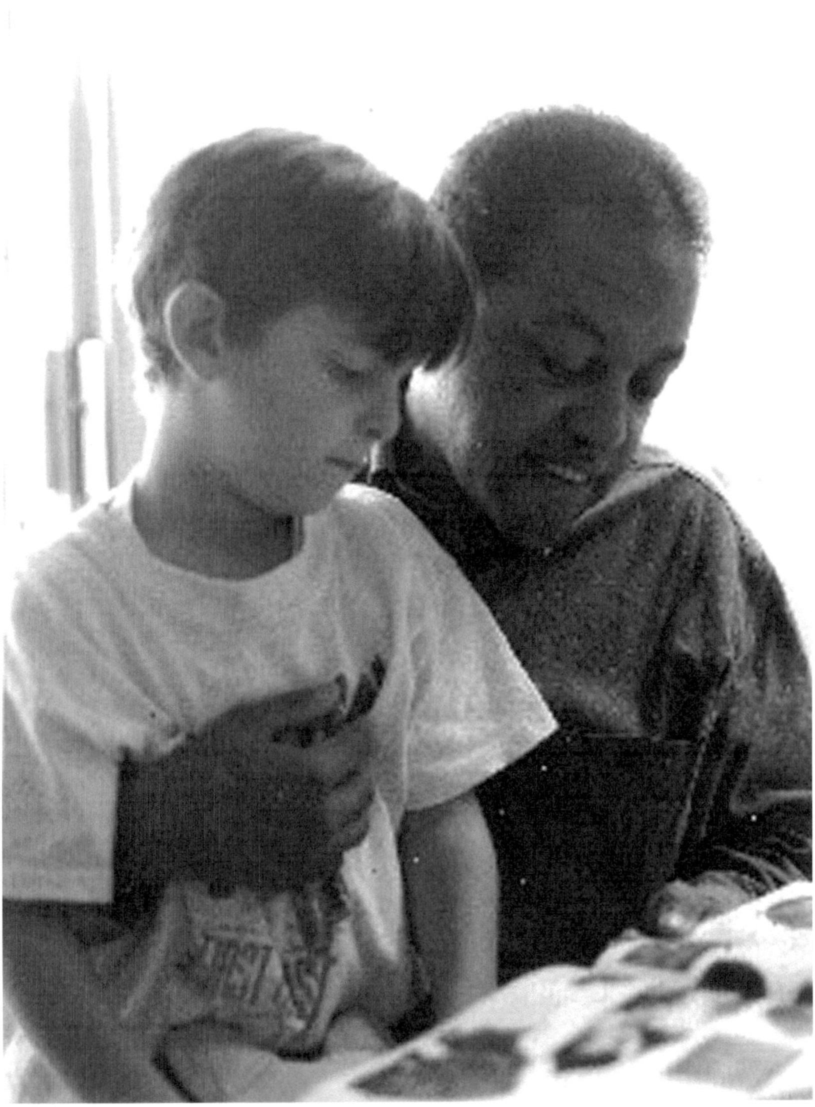

Figure 8.1. Ben Krause and Julius Scott, from memories written by Paul Krause, December 8, 2021, photograph courtesy of Paul Krause.

Yesterday's event [¡Presente!, December 13, 2021] was a needed gathering that served me and many others as restorative medicine in a difficult week. At Laurent's prompting, I managed to say a few thoughts near the end, and I tried to relate my visit with Julius and his parents at Hilton Head a few years back. After a wonderful lunch at their club, we went out to the deck, both father and

> son in their wheelchairs, and spent some time, sharing thoughts and gazing out over the vast Atlantic ocean towards the Caribbean and Africa.
>
> I'm afraid I choked up trying to describe an event that was so meaningful to all four of us. I felt a bit embarrassed, but it is probably good for all those younger folks to see an elder being at a loss for words. Afterwards, I recalled one other time where I surprised myself by being overcome with emotion when I was trying to say something brief and heartfelt. It was at the Highlander Center in Tennessee, when I was called upon suddenly to present a gift to Rosa Parks, whom I had never met. So it seems I only choke up for very special people.
>
> Lil and I are doing well, brightening our days by recalling so many different encounters with Julius, his love of the *Rockford Files*, and his wonderful turns of phrase. Yesterday, Lil remembered how, when tackling something difficult (or encouraging others to do likewise), he often observed, "Well, it sure beats cutting pulp wood!" What a special friend and inspiration for so many of us! (Peter Wood, December 14, 2021, Longmont, Colorado)

Peter also gave Julius a copy of his book, *Near Andersonville* (2010), which he dedicated: "To Julius S Scott, humanist, scholar, and special friend—with deep admiration and warmest best wishes for a fellow historian and member of the Dropping Canoe Society. Always, Peter H. Wood, October 2010."

Julius remembered Peter Wood as well, describing his essential assistance in helping Julius research connections between Black people in the Atlantic world:

> I wanted to know what one could say about the connections among Black people, about that particular relationship, to make Black people better understood. There were some particularly important things to understand about the connection between people in South Carolina and people in Barbados, for example, something that we learned about reading [my advisor] Peter Woods's book, *Black Majority: Negroes in Colonial South Carolina from 1670 through the Stono Rebellion* [1975]. You couldn't really understand the history of South Carolina without understanding how it was connected to Barbados. And even though Peter didn't know much about Barbados, he did know about South Carolina, so it kind of helped us to understand something about each of these places and the ways they tied in to other places connected to them.

That was something that was important to me. And I'm not sure why I went to graduate school when I felt ready to understand that question, but it was just by accident. The first semester in graduate school, I had to take two seminars, and the person who taught African American history was on leave. So Peter [Wood] said, "Look, you better find two other places besides Afro-America to focus on." So I said, "Well, I hadn't really done much work on, or enough work on, America in the 18th century. Therefore, I needed to really understand colonial and revolutionary North American, or what I thought was American, history."

I remember Professor Chuck Bergquist. He taught Modern Latin America, which I also took. And what ended up happening was, during the morning hours, when I had Peter's course, he talked about certain things in North America. And then in the afternoon, when we were in Professor Bergquist's course, we got a whole different view about areas of the world, really a different way of thinking about things. And honestly, my thing was, "Wow, we should do more thinking about the ways these places really connect to each other, as opposed to still thinking about them as separate and discrete areas."

The revolution in Haiti became an interesting way to do that. I was interested in the particulars of the revolution in Haiti, but the ways that connected to other things was what made it really interesting. I remember I went to Peter's class one day and he said, "You know what? Why don't you come give a guest lecture in my seminar? You can do it in a way that connects Haiti and the Haitian Revolution to the American Revolution. That would be really great."

So that was how these things accidentally connected for me (Connolly 2022).

Several of his colleagues and friends in the Departments of History; of Afroamerican and African Studies; and of Anthropology at the University of Michigan lamented Julius's passing as well.

I just learned of Julius's passing. I am devastated. He was a magnificent person and beloved by so many of us. (Sue Juster, December 6, 2021, Ann Arbor, Michigan)

We have been thinking of…the memories of Julius surge across the airwaves, including this morning's beautiful piece from the Associated Press in the *Miami Herald.* (Rebecca Scott, December 9, 2021, Ann Arbor, Michigan)

Although I had not seen Julius as much since he stopped teaching, I had always treasured him as a colleague. I invited him several times to talk to my students about Atlantic slavery and it was always so exciting. We had many long conversations about his dog (Moshie? [Mogie]) when he used to bring him by the department to visit with the staff, who universally loved Julius (and Moshie). Running into Julius in the hallway was always such a great pleasure. He was a remarkable person and I will miss him. I had just finished reviewing the Portuguese translation of Chapter 4 of Julius's book when I received word from Rebecca that he passed. The chapter is so spectacular and I was, once again, filled with admiration…Julius was treasured by so many of his colleagues. I'm very pleased that the possible translation and publication of his book in Brazil is moving forward. It will be a lovely tribute to him. (Sueann Caulfield, December 14, 2021, Ann Arbor, Michigan)

I was so terribly saddened to hear about Julius's passing. It's such an enormous loss for all of us who knew him and enjoyed his friendship, but for you and his family particularly so. Such a wonderful wonderful man—warm, funny, and deeply grounded in everything that mattered. (John Carson, December 7, 2021, Ann Arbor, Michigan)

Dr. Scott continued to shape our collective understanding of Atlantic history, slavery, the Haitian Revolution, and the lives and struggles of Black peoples from across the African diaspora—and jazz, always jazz—through classroom instruction, symposia, and conversations too numerous to count. His generosity with his time and insight was all the more remarkable given his many health challenges. (Angela Dillard, December 9, 2021, Ann Arbor, Michigan)

I am so sorry to hear about the passing of our beloved Julius this morning. This is very sad and an irreparable loss. May Julius's soul rest in peace. (Omolade Adunbi, December 6, 2023, Ann Arbor, Michigan)

… not sure how helpful I can be from a distance. Except to share that you are now even more in my thoughts … as is my enduring admiration for Julius. (James Chaffers, December 11, 2021, Ann Arbor, Michigan)

I am so heartbroken to hear this. He survived so much and we were so incredibly fortunate to have him in our lives. (Kelly Askew, December 6, 2021, Ann Arbor, Michigan)

We're so very sad and sorry to hear that his family and the world have lost Julius. What an incredible human being and brilliant mind he was, and on top of that, so courageous and forward-looking and funny and *present* despite the severe health challenges he faced for so long. How lucky we are to have had the privilege of knowing him. He fought so long and hard but we're glad he left peacefully. May his soul be showered with compassion. (Janet Richards and Stuart Kirsch, December 6, 2021, Ann Arbor, Michigan)

Staff members and physicians at the University of Michigan also sadly remembered Julius:

Julius was more than just a friend, he was a mentor to me. He helped guide me through my journey with diabetes and eventually with being a transplant recipient. We started working at UM the same year, and from that point on, he was someone I truly admired and appreciated for his brilliance and his humor. I don't think people realized how incredibly smart Julius was. We would share our prep school stories as well as swap musical stories—he was just naturally curious about all sorts of things, which of course, librarians like me understand completely. The ties were natural—my great-Grandmama was born in the same town as he was and we used to laugh about that a lot. I learned so much from him and now I try to urge current students in the same way he used to do—gently, with a deep passion for the African diaspora.

Even though we both were naughty and didn't always do what we should, we had an understanding that our bodies were dealing with issues that we had to accept and learn to cope with if we were going to continue. (Elizabeth James, August 31, 2022, Ann Arbor, Michigan)

I am heartbroken. I knew he was a giant as soon as we met but didn't know this other history. I'm truly sorry that I didn't get to celebrate his achievement with him. (Arno Kumagai, MD, December 18, 2021, Toronto, Canada)

The collaborators who worked with him on the publication of his book, *The Common Wind*, were also saddened.

Peter Wood just gave me the sad news. What a terrible loss, but what a life well lived. (Marcus Rediker, University of Pittsburgh, December 6, 2021, Pittsburgh, Pennsylvania)

Working with Julius was, without a doubt, the highlight of my half decade with Verso. He was so smart, humble, generous, and kind. That his work was

> taken up everywhere… is a testament to the undeniable power of his work. (Ben Mabie, Verso Press, December 15, 2021, Brooklyn, New York)

Last but not least, Julius's students—both graduates and undergraduates—had thoughtful memories of Julius.

> I first met Professor Scott in 2008, when I was myself a doctoral student at the University of Michigan. Julius, the man, remained easily accessible and unfailingly approachable, particularly to those who frequented Michigan's Center for Afroamerican and African Studies, as it was then known. But then there was "The Dissertation," often brought up in the form of a question: "Have you read The Dissertation?" Folks were referring to a nondescript tome with a faded blue binding, deep in the stacks and bursting with generations of accumulated marginalia. Graduate students took to making their mark in it, like a version of academic graffiti, perhaps befitting the hip-hop generation. Julius would no doubt improve upon my making such an easy cultural simile, as he was both a brilliant writer and a legendary lover of jazz. Still, students and faculty alike had granted him "battle-rapper" levels of street cred. His dissertation has been called "the most read, sought after and discussed English-language dissertation in the humanities and social sciences during the 20th century." Indeed, past students likened it to an underground mix tape. It had been swapped and trafficked to the point where mere citation counts could no longer do it justice. (Nathan Connolly, Johns Hopkins University, May 12, 2022, Baltimore, Maryland)
>
> I am so, so sorry to hear this news. Kelly sent me an email letting me know, and I am still processing this. Julius was a great mentor and teacher, and had a significant impact upon my trajectory as a graduate student at U of M. I will never forget how he stepped in to save the day at my defense when one of my committee members didn't show up. It was great seeing him recently when he came to the University of Pittsburgh in honor of his book, *The Common Wind.* He has truly left his mark in this world, and I am glad that he is no longer suffering. (Yolanda Covington, University of Massachusetts, Amherst, December 28, 2021)

A journal entry referred to Julius's action at Yolanda's defense: "Julius saved the day.… 'Be that,' he said, which was a reference to Omar Little in *The Wire*" (Journal, October 4, 2008).

As an undergraduate, Douglas Manigault took the introductory course for the Department of Afroamerican and African Studies (DAAS) at the University of Michigan, as he wrote:

> I just heard of Dr. Julius Scott's passing. I had the distinguished pleasure of taking AAS 111: Intro to Africa & Its Diaspora with Dr. Scott and Dr. Askew. Dr. Scott's passion for topics such as music, the Haitian revolution, and African culture was apparent. He was one of the reasons that I, as a freshman, decided to inquire, and ultimately attend, the abroad trip to Ghana. My memories of him are as long as my gratitude for him is. (Douglas F. Manigault III, December 13, 2021, Ann Arbor, Michigan)

This introductory course was taught by two DAAS faculty, one whose research focused on African American societies in the United States, Caribbean, and South America, while the other focused on Africa. When teaching this course, Julius introduced students to the practice of slavery in the United States and the Americas, the development of African American churches, abolition movements, the Haitian Revolution, and concepts of race. Along with other undergraduate and graduate courses, which included his course on John Coltrane, Julius had a remarkable teaching career at the University of Michigan.

George Streator and a Trip to the Woodlawn Cemetery

Julius had another project in mind after he completed his dissertation in 1986 that focused on the work of the African American writer, George Streator, whom Julius greatly admired. Beginning in 1933, Streator became a staff member of the National Association for the Advancement of Colored People (NAACP) and editor of its periodical, *The Crisis*, from which Julius made copious notes concerning Streator's union activities. Streator was also the first Black reporter who worked at the *New York Times*, beginning in 1945. He wrote numerous articles for the *Times* which focused on issues of racial discrimination and workers' rights. However, he was fired for editing articles "in order to present blacks in a more positive light." Yet the *Times* practiced racial discrimination: when the firm shifted to automatic elevators in 1961, "only eight of the forty-one displaced black elevator operators had been able to get better jobs elsewhere at the paper," what Streator referred to as the "Negro Removal Act" (see below). And in 1961, "the news department had one black copyeditor; there were two black reporters" (Tifft and Jones 1999: 277). After leaving the *Times* in 1949, George Streator became the editor of the journal, *The Pilot*.

Julius prepared two binder notebooks with photocopied articles written by Streator and extensive notes of Streator's correspondence with W. E. B. Du Bois and others. In one letter that Du Bois sent to Streator on April 17, 1935, Du Bois observed that "I have come to the conclusion that we have got to regard race prejudice in this country as fairly permanent for practical purposes" (Du Bois 1935). This view coincided with Streator's thinking, reflected in a letter to Norman M. Thomas, the leader of the US Socialist Party, written in 1933:

> I am calling on you as the best exponent of the Party to lay greater emphasis on the Negro and his plight. I wish I could hear an equivocating stand on racial justice by somebody speaking in the South. There is only one solid foundation for socialism in the South. It must begin with wiping out the color line in labor.... Again, I declare that the labor movement is the only answer, but the labor movement is mum as an old maid on the Negro question.[1]

Julius documented Streator's extensive work in detailing the situation of African American labor and what he referred to as discrimination under the "Negro Removal Act." In an article published on September 3, 1933 in *The Daily News*, Greensboro, North Carolina (which Julius photocopied), Streator (1933a) discusses a case in which a Black man who had worked for a business firm in Greensboro was suddenly fired:

> The most outrageous case of this kind that has come to public attention lately, however, is that of the Elm street firm which put in the street without notice a faithful employee of good record and long service on the flimsy grounds that the store did not have lavatory facilities to accommodate this single negro employee.... The firm in question could easily have created a job for the white man who now serves this store as porter... The colored man now walking the street will not effect an adjustment to the change very easily (Streator 1933a).

[1] Letter from George Streator to Norman Thomas, September 13, 1933, New York Public Library, from typed excerpt in Julius Scott's notebook (Streator 1933b).

Surely, Julius found this story about separate bathroom facilities reminiscent of his own experience in the first grade at MacGregor Elementary School in Houston.

Streator wrote an article entitled, "Negro Doctor, 81, 'Oldest' Yet Active," for the *New York Times*. The doctor, Eugene Percy Roberts, was also one of the founders of the St. James Presbyterian Church, which is now located in Harlem. It is presently a Historic African American Congregation of the Presbyterian Church (USA) ("One Hundred and 127 years and counting!"). Yet:

> Dr. Roberts said that there is a tendency here to list "too many Negro firsts, the community forgetting that the Negro citizens with their ups and downs have been active for many years in civic affairs, and frequently been accorded due recognition" (Streator 1949)

Dr. Roberts' observation is related to a comment that Julius made when he was interviewed by Dr. Caroline Lattimore in 1991. Julius, who achieved several integration firsts, made a similar observation in his interview with Dr. Lattimore: "We love superstars but you don't have to be a superstar to accomplish current history." In other words, much attention has been given to prominent Blacks in US society, whereas many Black people have contributed to civil rights and equality in their country and communities.

Julius's admiration for George Streator led him to visit his gravesite in the Woodlawn Cemetery in the Bronx, New York, in June 2012 (Figure 8.2). "He went up to the Bronx, it was fine, a long subway ride but no problems. Julius found the Streator grave which was far, far from the entrance. They had someone from security take him" (Journal, June 4, 2012).

It is unfortunate that Julius was unable to create the manuscript he intended to write as surprisingly little has been written explicitly about George Streator. And it would have been particularly appropriate, unfortunately, as Streator would have been appalled by the current situation in the United States. Attempts to support various forms of White supremacy in the United States of America have led some politicians to undermine the teaching of African American history, which could omit learning about the murder of Emmett Till for whom a national monument was recently created (Green 2023). It also led some to suggest that "slaves developed skills which, in some instances, could be applied for their personal benefit," a statement which has

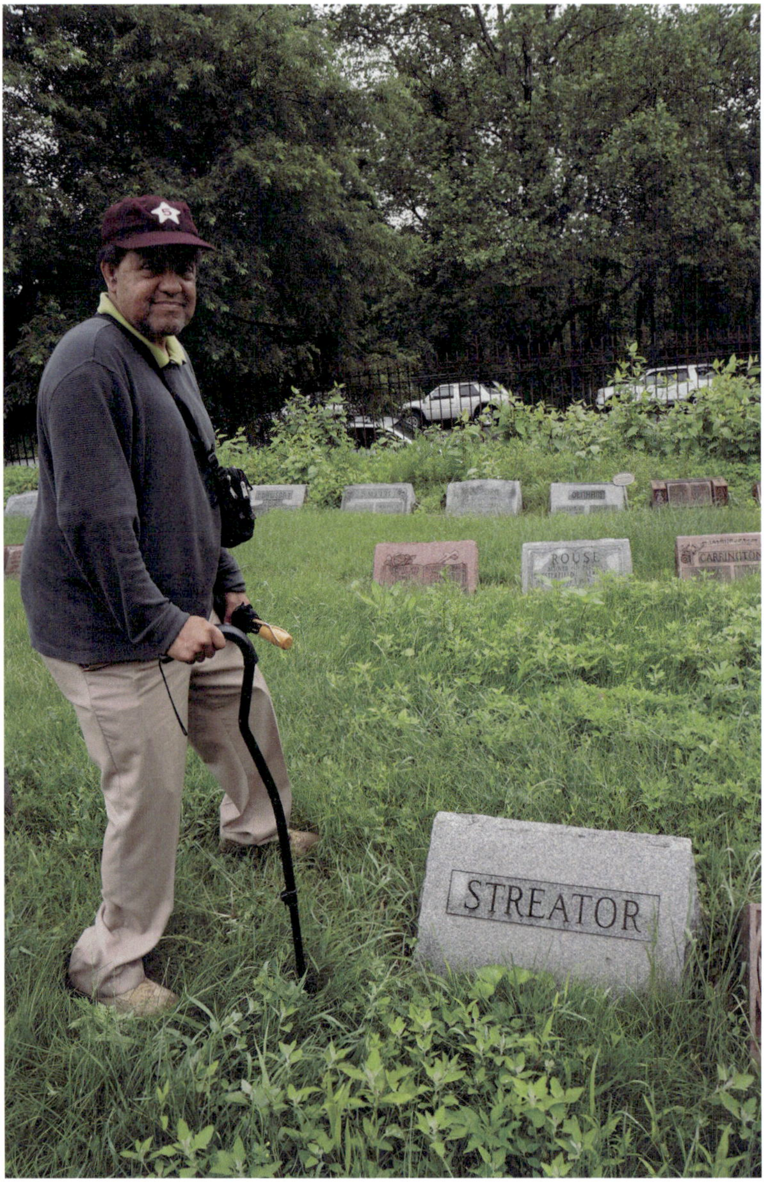

Figure 8.2. George Streator grave, Woodlawn Cemetery, the Bronx, New York City, June 4, 2012; photograph by E.P. Renne.

appalled many. It would have appalled Julius in its intention to put "a more pleasant sheen" on slavery in the United States (Bouie 2023). Nonetheless, being Julius Scott, he would have preferred a more complicated, historical interpretation.

Bibliography

Primary Sources

Breeden, Edwin. 2017. *Educational Politics and the Making of School Desegregation Policy in Houston, Texas*. PhD dissertation, Department of History, Rice University, Houston, Texas. https://hdl.handle.net/1911/105625.

Connolly, Nathan. 2022. "An Uncommon, Unconquerable Mind: Our Friend, Julius S. Scott III (1955–2021)." *Public Books*, May 12, 2022. https://www.publicbooks.org/julius-s-scott-iii-1955-2021-the-common-wind.

Dubois, Laurent. 2021. "Julius S. Scott: ¡Presente!, Zoom Memorial." December 13, 2021.

Du Bois, W. E. B. "Letter from W. E. B. Du Bois to George Streator, April 17, 1935." W. E. B. Du Bois Papers (MS 312). Special Collections and University Archives, University of Massachusetts Amherst Libraries. https://credo.library.umass.edu/view/full/mums312-b076-i210.

Lord Kitchener. 2004. "If You're Brown," KM Records (released 1 August).

MacGregor Elementary School website, Houston. https://www.houstonisd.org/macgregores.

Mayo Clinic. 2022. "Coronary Artery Bypass Grafting Surgery." www.mayoclinic.org/tests-procedures/coronary-bypass-surgery/about/pac-20384589.

Mayo Clinic. 2023. "Type 1 Diabetes." www.mayoclinic.org/diseases-conditions/type-1-diabetes/symptoms-causes/syc-20353011.

Mineo, Liz. 2022. "Celebrating the Founder of Black History Month." Interview: Jarvis Givens. *The Harvard Gazette*, February 1, 2022. https://news.harvard.edu/gazette/story/2022/02/celebrating-black-history-months-founder.

Oyez. 2003. "Grutter vs. Bollinger," 539 U.S. 306 (2003). https://www.oyez.org/cases/2002/02-241.

Renne, Elisha. 1999–2021. Journals, unpublished.

Ross, Delores et al. v. Houston Independent School District, et al., No. 81-2323 (5th Cir. 1983). *Open Jurist*. https://openjurist.org/699/f2d/218/ross-v-houston-independent-school-district

Scott, Julius S. 1986. *The Common Wind: Afro-American Currents in the Age of the Haitian Revolution*. PhD dissertation, Department of History, Duke University.

Scott, Julius. 2017. "A LOVE SUPREME: John Coltrane, the Sixties, and 'Jazz'", Syllabus. Department of History, University of Michigan, Fall 2017.

St. Andrew By-the-Sea, United Methodist Church. 2022. Program for the Memorial Service for Dr. Julius S. Scott, III. Hilton Head Island, South Carolina, February 5, 2022.

Streator, George. 1933b. Letter to Norman Thomas, September 13, 1933. New York: New York Public Library.

Book reviews

Bartlett, Tom. 2018. "An Underground Sensation Arrives: The Three-Decade Publication Saga of a Revered Manuscript." *The Chronicle Review*, November 2, 2018. https://www.chronicle.com/article/An-underground-sensation/245000.

Bell, David. 2019. "The Contagious Revolution." *New York Review of Books*, December 19, 2019. https://www.nybooks.com/articles/2019/12/19/the-contagious-revolution-haiti.

Bhatia, Pooja. 2020. "The End of the Plantocracy." *London Review of Books*, November 19, 2020, 21–23.

Bressler, Malkah. 2019. "Currents of Revolution: On Julius S. Scott's 'The Common Wind'." *LA Review of Books*, March 21, 2019. https://lareviewofbooks.org/article/currents-of-revolution-on-julius-s-scotts-the-common-wind.

Hazareesingh, Sudhir. 2019. "Masterless People." *Times Literary Supplement*, March 15, 2019, 36–37.

Parker, Gregory. 2019. "Celebrating Julius S. Scott's *The Common Wind*: Landmark Dissertation Published After 30 Years." *University of Michigan History Department Newsletter*. https://lsa.umich.edu/history/news-events/all-news/facultynews/celebrating-julius-s--scott-s-the-common-wind.html.

Sinha, Manisha. 2019. "The Mobile Resistance." *The Nation*, June 3/10, 35–37.

Interviews

Connolly, Nathan. 2021. Interview: Julius Scott, on Atlantic history. Ann Arbor, Michigan, March 2021.

Lattimore, Caroline. 1991. Interview: Julius Scott, "In Times Like These," about Black History Month. Durham, North Carolina, 1991.

Renne, Elisha. 2019a. Interview: Julius Scott, about his dog, Mogie. Ann Arbor, Michigan, November 30, 2019.

Renne, Elisha. 2019b. Interview: Julius Scott, about his primary school education. Ann Arbor, Michigan, December 22, 2019.

Renne, Elisha. 2021. Interview: Ann Scott, February 5, 2021.

Renne, Elisha. 2022. Interview: Ann Scott, about Julius Scott's education, health. Hilton Head, South Carolina, November 22, 2022.

Secondary Sources

Abi-Habib, Maria, Natalie Kitroeff, Frances Robles and Nick Madigan. 2023. "U.S. Arrests Four More in the Assassination of Haiti's President." *New York Times*, February 14, 2023. https://www.nytimes.com/2023/02/14/world/americas/haiti-president-assassination-americans.html.

Anonymous. 1972. "230 Vying for Merit Scholarships." *Birmingham Post-Herald*, September14, 1972, 32.

Bouie, Jamelle. 2023. "In Lessons on Slavery, Context Matters." *New York Times*, July 29, 2023. https://www.nytimes.com/2023/07/29/opinion/florida-schools-history-slavery.html.

Braudel, Fernand. 1972. *The Mediterranean and the Mediterranean World in the Age of Philip II*. Translated by Siân Reynolds. New York: Harper & Row.

Bryant, Salatheia. 2004. "Integration Did Not Come to HISD Until 1984." *Houston Chronicle*, May 16, 2004 (updated July 12, 2011). https://www.chron.com/news/houston-texas/article/Integration-did-not-come-to-HISD-until-1984-1512348.php.

Bullwinkle Studios LLC. 2014. *Mr. Peabody and Sherman*. Costa Mesa, California: Jay Ward Productions, Inc.

Crowley, Michael, Michael Shear, and Eric Schmitt. 2021. "Biden Administration Shows Little Appetite for Haiti's Troop Request." *New York Times*, July 10, 2021 (updated 13 July). https://www.nytimes.com/2021/07/10/us/politics/biden-haiti-troop-request.html.

Downey, Maureen. 2019. "These Students Walked Onto Westminster Campus and Into History." *The Atlanta Journal-Constitution,* January 9, 2019. https://www.ajc.com/blog/get-schooled/these-students-walked-onto-westminster-campus-and-intohistory/zZt776u8nu5mDMPi9jyIUJ.

Dubois, Laurent, and Julius Scott, eds. 2010. *The Origins of the Black Atlantic*. Routledge: New York and London.

Encyclopedia Britannica. 2023. "Haiti and the Haitian Revolution." https://www.britannica.com/place/Haiti/The-Haitian-Revolution.

Equiano, Olaudah. 1987. *The Interesting Narrative of the Life of Olaudah Equiano, or Gustavus Vassa, the African, Written by Himself*. In *The Classic Slave Narratives*, edited by Henry Louis Gates, Jr., 1–182. New York and London: Penguin.

Gamio, Lazaro, Constant Méheut, Catherine Porter, Selam Gebrekidan, Allison McCann, and Matt Apuzzo. 2022. "Haiti's Lost Billions." *New York Times*, May 20, 2022. https://www.nytimes.com/interactive/2022/05/20/world/americas/enslaved-haiti-debt-timeline.html.

Garragus, John D. 2006. *Before Haiti: Race and Citizenship in French Saint-Domingue*. New York: Palgrave Macmillan.

Gebrekidan, Selam, Matt Apuzzo, Catherine Porter and Constant Méheut. 2022. "Invade Haiti, Wall Street Urged. U.S. Obliged." *New York Times*, May 20, 2022 (updated May 26, 2022). https://www.nytimes.com/2022/05/20/world/haiti-wall-street-us-banks.html.

Girard, Philippe. 2020. "Isaac Sasportas, the 1799 Slave Conspiracy in Jamaica, and Sephardic Ties to the Haitian Revolution." *Jewish History* 33: 403–35.

Givens, Jarvis R. 2021. *Fugitive Pedagogy: Carter G. Woodson and the Art of Black Teaching.* Cambridge: Harvard University Press.

Green, Erica. 2023. "Biden Creates Monument to Emmett Till Amid Fights Over Black History." *New York Times*, July 25, 2023. https://www.nytimes.com/2023/07/21/us/desantis-florida-black-history-standards.html.

Hill, Jane H. 2008. *The Everyday Language of White Racism*. Chichester, UK; Malden, MA: Wiley-Blackwell.

Jackson, Melvin. 1969. *Privateers in Charleston, 1793-1796: An Account of a French Palatinate in South Carolina*. Washington, D.C.: Smithsonian Institution Press.

James, Winston. 2010. *The Struggles of John Brown Russwurm: The Life and Writings of a Pan-Africanist Pioneer, 1799-1851*. New York: New York University Press.

Kellar, William. 1999. *Make Haste Slowly: Moderates, Conservatives, and School Desegregation in Houston*. College Station: Texas A&M University Press.

Kluger, Richard. 2004. *Simple Justice: The History of Brown v. Board of Education and Black America's Struggle for Equality*, revised, expanded. New York: Knopf.

Kuethe, Allan J. 1978. *Military Reform and Society in New Grenada, 1773-1808*. Gainesville: University Presses of Florida.

Maloney, Jim. 1961. "District Absentee Policy is Voted Down by Board," *Houston Chronicle*, October 22, 1961.

Matthews, David, Sue Beatty, Pam Dyson, Laurie King, Niki Meston, Aparna Pal, and Jenny Shaw. 2008. *Diabetes*. Oxford: Oxford University Press.

McCollum, Brian. 2017. "Detroit Jazz Festival Unveils 2017 Artist Lineup." *Detroit Free Press*, April 19, 2017. https://www.freep.com/story/entertainment/music/2017/04/19/detroit-jazz-festival-unveils-2017-artist-lineup/100641320/.

McGowen, Ninian. 1961. "School Bd Refuses to Hear Minister." *Houston Chronicle*, October 1961.

Méheut, Constant, and Catherine Porter. 2023. "Macron Honors Haitian Revolutionary, But Leaves Much Unsaid." *New York Times*, April 28, 2023. https://www.nytimes.com/2023/04/27/world/europe/macron-toussaint-louverture-speech.html.

Melish, Joanne Pope. 1998. *Disowning Slavery: Gradual Emancipation and "Race" in New England, 1780-1860*. Ithaca NY: Cornell University Press.

Mervosh, Sarah. 2023. "DeSantis Faces Swell of Criticism Over Florida's New Standards for Black History." *New York Times*, July 21, 2023. https://www.nytimes.com/2023/07/21/us/desantis-florida-black-history-standards.html.

Nagourney, Eric. 2022. "6 Takeaways About Haiti's Reparations to France." *New York Times*, May 20, 2022. https://www.nytimes.com/2022/05/20/world/americas/takeaways-haiti-reparations-france.html.

Patel, Vimal. 2023. "At UChicago, a Debate Over Free Speech and Cyber Bullying." *New York Times*, July 3, 2023. https://www.nytimes.com/2023/07/03/us/university-of-chicago-whiteness-free-speech.html.

Polgreen, Lydia. 2022. "'This Is It. This Is Our Chance.' It's Time For Everyone to Get Out of Haiti's Way." *New York Times*, October 12, 2022. https://www.nytimes.com/2022/10/12/opinion/haiti-montana-accords-reparations.html.

Porter, Catherine, Constant Méheut, Selam Gebrekidan, and Matt Apuzzo. 2022a. "The Ransom: A Look Under the Hood." *New York Times*, May 20, 2022 (updated May 22, 2022). https://www.nytimes.com/2022/05/20/world/americas/haiti-bibliography.html.

Porter, Catherine, Constant Méheut, Matt Apuzzo, and Selam Gebrekidan. 2022b. "The Roots of Haiti's Misery: Reparation to Enslavers." *New York Times*, May 20, 2022 (updated November 16, 2022). https://www.nytimes.com/2022/05/20/world/americas/haiti-history-colonized-france.html.

Purdy, Michelle A. 2018. *Transforming the Elite: Black Students and the Desegregation of Private Schools*. Chapel Hill: University of North Carolina Press.

Rediker, Marcus. 2018. "Foreword." In Julius Scott, *The Common Wind: Afro-American Currents in the Age of the Haitian Revolution*. London, New York: Verso, ix–xiii.

Riskin, Jessica. 2023. "The Poisonous Legacy." *New York Review of Books*, June 22, 2023, 34–36.

Roberts, Sam. 2021. "Julius S. Scott, Groundbreaking Historian of the Caribbean, Dies at 66." *New York Times*, December 16, 2021. https://www.nytimes.com/2021/12/16/obituaries/julius-scott-dead-common-wind.html.

Russwurm, John. 2010. "The Condition and Prospects of Hayti." In Winston James, *The Struggles of John Brown Russwurm: The Life and Writings of a Pan-Africanist Pioneer, 1799-1851*. New York: New York University Press, 131–34.

Saul, Stephanie. 2022. "Affirmative action was banned at two top universities. They say they need it." *New York Times*, 26 August. https://www.nytimes.com/2022/08/26/us/affirmative-action-admissions-supreme-court.html.

Schlesinger, Benjamin. 1967. "The Jews of Jamaica: A Historical View." *Caribbean Quarterly* 13: 46.

Scott, Julius S. 2018. *The Common Wind: Afro-American Currents in the Age of the Haitian Revolution*. London, New York: Verso.

Shange, Ntozake. 1997. "Toussaint Louverture." In *For Colored Girls Who Have Considered Suicide/When the Rainbow Is Enuf*. New York: Scribner, pp. 32–35.

Streator, George. 1933a. "The NRA and Fairness." *The Daily News*, Greensboro, September 3, 1933.

Streator, George. 1949. "Negro Doctor, 81, 'Oldest,' Yet Active." *New York Times*, April 7, 1949.

Sullivan, Eileen, and Steve Fisher. 2023. "At the End of a Hard Journey, Migrants Face Another: Navigating Bureaucracy." *New York Times*, March 10, 2023. https://www.nytimes.com/2023/03/10/us/politics/migrants-asylum-biden-mexico.html.

Tifft, Susan, and Alex Jones. 1999. *The Trust: The Private and Powerful Family Behind the New York Times*. Boston: Little, Brown and Company.

von Humboldt, Alexander. 1970. *Relation Historique Du Voyage Aux Régions Équinoxiales du Nouveau Continent*, 3 vols. Stuttgart: F.A. Brockhaus.

Wood, Peter. 1975. *Black Majority: Negroes in Colonial South Carolina From 1670 Through the Stono Rebellion*. New York: Norton.

Wood, Peter. 2010. *Near Andersonville: Winslow Homer's Civil War*. Cambridge, MA: Harvard University Press.

Woodson, Carter G. 1922. *The Negro in Our History*, 7th edition. Washington, D.C.: The Associated Publishers, Inc.